Health Informatics

(formerly Computers in Health Care)

Kathryn J. Hannah   Marion J. Ball
Series Editors

Springer

New York
Berlin
Heidelberg
Hong Kong
London
Milan
Paris
Tokyo

Health Informatics Series
(formerly Computers in Health Care)

Series Editors
Kathryn J. Hannah   Marion J. Ball

(continued after index)

Rosemary Nelson   Marion J. Ball
Editors

Consumer Informatics
*Applications and Strategies in
Cyber Health Care*

With 23 Illustrations

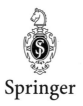

Springer

Rosemary Nelson, RN, BC,
CPHIMS, FHIMSS
President and CEO
MDM Strategies, Inc.
Merritt Island FL 32952 and
Adjunct Faculty
Johns Hopkins University
School of Nursing
Baltimore, MD 21205, USA

Marion J. Ball, EdD
Vice President, Clinical Solutions
Healthlink, Inc.
Baltimore, MD 21210 and
Adjunct Professor
Johns Hopkins University
School of Nursing
Baltimore, MD 21205, USA

Series Editors:

Kathryn J. Hannah, PhD, RN
Adjunct Professor, Department
  of Community Health Science
Faculty of Medicine
The University of Calgary
Calgary, Alberta, T2N 4N1 Canada

Marion J. Ball, EdD
Vice President, Clinical Solutions
Healthlink, Inc.
Baltimore, MD 21210 and
Adjunct Professor
Johns Hopkins University
School of Nursing
Baltimore, MD 21205, USA

Cover illustration by Roy Wiemann, 2003.

Library of Congress Cataloging-in-Publication Data
Nelson, Rosemary
    Consumer informatics : applications and strategies in cyber health care / Rosemary
  Nelson, Marion Ball.
      p. cm – (Health informatics)
    Includes index.
    ISBN 0-387-40414-7 (alk. paper)
      1. Medical informatics.   2. Internet.   3. Telecommunicatioin medicine.
    4. Information storage and retrieval systems—Medicine.   5. Consumer education.
  I. Ball, Marion J. II. Title. III. Series.
  R858.N45 2004
  025.06´61—dc21

ISBN 0-387-40414-7   Printed on acid-free paper.

Printed in the United States of America.   (KP/EB)

9 8 7 6 5 4 3 2 1   SPIN   10938539

Springer-Verlag is a part of *Springer Science+Business Media*

springeronline.com

Series Preface

This series is directed to healthcare professionals who are leading the transformation of health care by using information and knowledge. Launched in 1988 as Computers in Health Care, the series offers a broad range of titles: some addressed to specific professions such as nursing, medicine, and health administration; others to special areas of practice such as trauma and radiology. Still other books in the series focus on interdisciplinary issues, such as the computer-based patient record, electronic health records, and networked healthcare systems.

Renamed Health Informatics in 1998 to reflect the rapid evolution in the discipline now known as health informatics, the series will continue to add titles that contribute to the evolution of the field. In the series, eminent experts, serving as editors or authors, offer their accounts of innovations in health informatics. Increasingly, these accounts go beyond hardware and software to address the role of information in influencing the transformation of healthcare delivery systems around the world. The series also increasingly focuses on "peopleware" and the organizational, behavioral, and societal changes that accompany the diffusion of information technology in health services environments.

These changes will shape health services in this new millennium. By making full and creative use of the technology to tame data and to transform information, health informatics will foster the development of the knowledge age in health care. As coeditors, we pledge to support our professional colleagues and the series readers as they share advances in the emerging and exciting field of health informatics.

Kathryn J. Hannah
Marion J. Ball

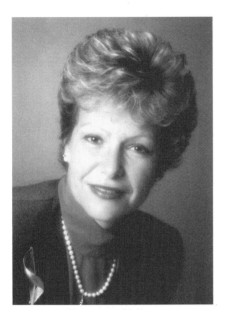

Rosemary Nelson

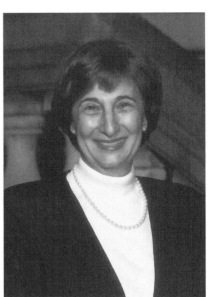

Marion J. Ball

Preface

More than 70 million Americans have used the Internet to research health issues, and, according to a December 2002 survey from the Pew Research Center, 6 million go online each day to get health information. The Pew survey indicates that, with more than 100,000 active health information Web sites, two thirds to 80% of consumers feel they can filter the information to get what they want. A similar study conducted in 2001 by the U.S. Department of Commerce (DOC) indicates that 75% of U.S. households with annual incomes of at least $50,000 a year have access to the Internet, while another DOC study, conducted in 2002, demonstrates that 34.9% of U.S. consumers seek information online about health services or medical practices. To substantiate further the consumer's passion with online health services, a survey conducted by Cyber Dialogue in May 2000, which focused on who consumers trust online, shows that consumers trust their own doctors first (62%), followed by national experts (61%), followed by online information posted by hospitals (58%). Other research reflects that as many as one third of all queries to major Internet search engines are health related, covering all aspects of healthcare delivery, disease management, medications, herbal therapies, and home treatment alternatives.

These statistics are indicative not only of the pervasiveness of the Internet in consumers' quests for healthcare information but also of their reliance on the accuracy of that information. These attitudes also reflect the characteristic of a dominant group of today's population—Baby Boomers and Generation Xers—who are health conscious, technologically savvy, and who do not readily accept the status quo. These trends are expected to continue and expand as the Baby Boomers age. At the same time, healthcare providers continue to harness the capabilities of the Internet, creating new opportunities and new paradigms for the delivery of healthcare information, and, most importantly, for the delivery of health care itself.

Consumer empowerment and active interaction between consumers and the Internet is a trend that was foreseen as early as a decade ago, in 1993, by Dr. Thomas Ferguson. A pioneering physician, author, and researcher, Ferguson has been studying and writing about the empowered medical consumer since 1975, and about online health resources for consumers since 1987. In 1993, Ferguson and several other early pioneers who were developing information technology (IT) systems designed for use by healthcare consumers organized a conference sponsored by Healthwise Inc. and the National Wellness Association. The conference, *Consumer Health Informatics: Bringing the Patient Into the Loop*, took place on July 16-18, 1993, in Stevens Point, Wisconsin, and reflected the first appearance of the term *consumer health informatics* in both the conference brochure and the proceedings. Needless to say, the topic generated nationwide interest, and at the 1993 annual meeting of the American Medical Informatics Association (AMIA), Ferguson and Dr. Warner Slack presented a half-day tutorial, entitled, "Consumer Health Informatics: Bringing the Patient into the Loop," in which they discussed the advent of IT systems specifically designed for use by healthcare consumers. At the time, Ferguson proposed that a role change was in the offing in the physician–patient encounter. Whereas in the past the physician had taken on a role of authority and the patient one of compliance, Ferguson posited that in the future the physician's role would be more like that of "tech support," where the customer describes the problem to be fixed, articulates the desirable result, and reports when satisfaction has been achieved. In describing this scenario, Ferguson became the first to coin the term *consumer health informatics*, as reflected in the AMIA records. The first AMIA publication on consumer health informatics was the manual that Ferguson and Slack prepared for the 1993 AMIA tutorial. Since that time, other national associations and conferences, such as the Healthcare Information and Management Systems Society and the National Managed Health Care Congress, have sponsored education sessions focused on bringing patients, their families and friends, and consumers in general "into the loop" via information, technology, and virtual communities.

The result of these efforts has been a paradigm shift that now makes this book a necessity for both those *providing* and those *seeking* healthcare information on the Internet. As such, this book is of interest to healthcare administrators, IT professionals, and healthcare practitioners. It is also an invaluable tool in healthcare informatics training programs, for no development occurs today where informaticians are not concerned. Finally, it also speaks to consumers determined to seek empowerment within the healthcare system.

As expert healthcare informaticians, the editors of this volume have structured it to explore those technology-enabled applications that may very well become the cornerstones of our evolving healthcare systems. Woven through the volume is also an emphasis on the empowerment of all involved, whether they are healthcare professionals, laypersons, or consumer recipients of health care. Each chapter describes the role of computers, technology, and telecommunications (CTT) as enablers within a specific application focused on consumers' needs. These applications empower professionals in their efforts to serve those who are ill and those who are well. The applications are also ones that empower consumers as they seek information, analyze their unique healthcare needs, and make decisions about their own health. By focusing on empowerment in the service of health for all, the book illustrates the issues raised by consumer informatics through actual examples. Whether addressing disease management, bioterrorism surveillance/detection, or traveler health, the contributors illustrate how CTT can strengthen the human element in health care.

More specifically, the book utilizes both applied use and pragmatic examples to address the information needs of patients and consumers in three distinct areas: collaborative healthware, research and development, and telemedicine and telehealth. An introduction to each section provides the context for the applications presented in the individual chapters and in addition highlights other issues and areas not covered in the volume. In the sections and actual applications described, the technology is presented as an enabler, and the authors, therefore, provide greater focus on business practices, consumers' acceptance, use of the technology, and policy issues.

Section I, for example, defines collaborative healthware and explains why this is the next compelling step for consumer health informatics. In collaborative health care, cooperation among stakeholders will allow health systems to do business in different ways. Four chapters show how this approach is currently being applied in diverse settings. Examples include the management and empowerment of vulnerable populations; a patient-centric Web-based system that allows secure messaging and allows patients to schedule appointments, order prescription refills, and interact with their own medical records; a Web-based information and support system for patient home recovery after surgery; and a statewide effort in the care of elderly patients that utilizes a virtual hospital and virtual nurse visits at home.

Section II addresses initiatives under development that include the use of CTT to support public health and biodefense and disaster management; to set standards of quality for information found on the Internet; and to provide secure access to computerized patient records.

Section III presents a panoramic view of the interactive use of telemedicine and the consumer in disease management, home telehealth, online communities, and computer-consumer interviewing. New educational paradigms, such as distance learning for medical, nursing, and online consumer communities, are also discussed.

The authors and editors recognize that we are only at the early stages of realizing the value that consumer health informatics can offer to consumers and the population at large. Broader understanding of consumers' expectations and broader dissemination of the technology will lead to second-level benefits that can include design and implementation of public health interventions, improving population health, and evaluating the use of these technologies. According to a 2002 Harris Survey, 90% of U.S. adults who use the Internet would like to be able to e-mail their physicians to ask whether or not a visit is necessary (77%); schedule appointments (71%); refill prescriptions (71%); and receive the results of medical tests (70%). More than a third stated that they would be willing to pay out-of-pocket for the ability to communicate online with their physicians. More than half said they would be influenced to choose a doctor or a health plan that offers online patient services over one that does not. Many physicians have concluded that communicating with patients online offers as many benefits to providers as it does to patients. A recent Healtheon survey found that 33% of physicians have begun communicating with patients by e-mail, up from an estimated 1% to 2% only 2 years earlier.

Consumers are *demanding* that we capitalize on the use of CTT to service their healthcare needs. We challenge you, our readers, to join us in taking consumer health informatics to the next level. We hope you enjoy this book!

Rosemary Nelson
Marion J. Ball

Acknowledgments

Numerous clinical and healthcare informatics experts have contributed to the writing and editing of this book, which responds to current driving forces and emerging approaches in consumer informatics. This book represents the collective clinical, research, and informatics viewpoints of our healthcare industry and addresses the growing needs of consumers in healthcare services.

We extend special thanks to the following individuals for dedicating their time, energy, and enthusiasm to this project. Their many hours of research, writing, and reviewing have made this book a reality: Judy Douglas, Johns Hopkins University School of Nursing; Robert Fromberg, Healthcare Financial Management Association; Dr. Edward Martin, Science Applications International Corporation; Norris Orms, Healthcare Information and Management Systems Society; Stacey Prus, Healthcare Information and Management Systems Society; and Dr. Charles Safran, Clinician Support Technology.

Rosemary Nelson
Marion J. Ball

Contents

SECTION I COLLABORATIVE HEALTHWARE

SECTION II RESEARCH AND DEVELOPMENT

SECTION III TELEMEDICINE AND TELEHEALTH

Contributors

Ron D. Appel, PhD
Professor, Swiss Institute of Bioinformatics, University Hospital of Geneva and University of Geneva, Geneva, Switzerland

Dixie B. Baker, PhD
Corporate President for Technology, CTO, Enterprise and Health Solutions, Science Applications International Corporation, San Diego, CA 92121, USA

Marion J. Ball, EdD
Vice President, Clinical Informatics Strategies, Healthlink Inc., Baltimore, MD 21210; Adjunct Professor, Johns Hopkins University School of Nursing, Baltimore, MD 21205, USA

Celia Boyer
Executive Director, Health on the Net Foundation (HON), Geneva University Hospitals, DIM, Geneva, Switzerland

Patricia Flatley Brennan, RN, PhD, FAAN
Moehlman Bascom Professor, University of Wisconsin-Madison, Madison, WI 53792, USA

M. Kay Cresci, PhD, RN, APRN, BC
Assistant Professor, Johns Hopkins University School of Nursing, Baltimore, MD 21205, USA

Patrice Degoulet, MD, PhD
Professor of Medical Informatics, Broussais Faculty of Medicine, Paris VI University, Paris, France

Katharina V. Echt, PhD
Health Research Scientist, Atlanta VA Medical Center, Rehabilitation Research & Development Center, Emory University Center for Health in Aging, Atlanta, GA 30322, USA

Victoria Elfrink, RN(c), PhD
Director, Consumer Informatics, iTelehealth Inc., Frederick, MD 21702, USA

David Ellis
Editor and Publisher, *Health Futures Digest*, Lansing, MI 48933, USA

Marius Fieschi, MD, PhD
Professor of Medical Informatics, Faculty of Medicine, University of Aix-Marseille II, Marseille, France

Denise Goldsmith, RN, MPH
Director, Clinical Informatics, Clinician Support Technology, One Wells Avenue, Newton, MA 02459, USA

John D. Halamka, MD, MS
Chief Information Officer, Harvard Medical School; Chief Medical Information Officer, CareGroup HealthCare System, Boston, MA 02120, USA

Marie-Christine Jaulent, PhD
Head, Health Knowledge Engineering Library, Broussais Faculty of Medicine, Paris VI University, Paris, France

Josette Jones, RN, PhD, BC
Assistant Professor, School of Nursing – School of Informatics, Indiana University, Purdue University Indianapolis, Indianapolis, IN 46202-5143, USA

Michael G. Kienzle, MD
Associate Dean for Clinical Affairs and Biomedical Communications, College of Medicine, University of Iowa; Chief Technology Officer, University of Iowa Health Care, Iowa City, IA 52242, USA

Edward D. Martin, MD
Sector Vice President, Science Applications International Corporation, San Diego, CA 92121, USA

Daniel Masys, MD, FACP
Director of Biomedical Informatics, Professor of Medicine, University of California, San Diego School of Medicine, San Diego, CA 92103-8811, USA

Joël Ménard, MD
Professor of Public Health, Broussais Faculty of Medicine, Paris VI University, Paris, France

Ronald C. Merrell, MD, FACS
Stuart McGuire Professor and Chairman, Department of Surgery, Virginia Commonwealth University, Richmond, VA 23298-0645, USA

Shirley M. Moore, RN, PhD
Case Western Reserve University, Cleveland, OH 44106, USA

Roger W. Morrell, PhD
Director of Research, GeroTech Corporation, Reston, VA 20191, USA

Rosemary Nelson, RN, Colonel, AN (ret.)
President and CEO, MDM Strategies, Inc., Merritt Island, FL 32952, and Adjunct Faculty, Johns Hopkins University School of Nursing, Baltimore, MD 21205, USA

John S. Parker, MD; Major General, MC (ret.)
Senior Vice President, Enterprise and Health Solutions Sector, Science Applications International Corp, San Diego, CA 92121, USA

Charles Safran, MD
Chairman and Chief Executive Officer, Clinician Support Technology, One Wells Avenue, Newton, MA 02459, USA

Daniel Z. Sands, MD, MPH
Assistant Professor of Medicine, Harvard Medical School, Clinical Systems Integration Architect, Beth Israel Deaconess Medical Center, Boston, MA 02215, USA

Loretta Schlachta-Fairchild, PhD, CHE
President & CEO, iTelehealth Inc., Frederick, MD 21702, USA

Jeffrey A. Spaeder, MD
Fellow in Cardiology, Johns Hopkins University School of Medicine, Baltimore, MD 21205, USA

Connie Visovsky, RN, PhD
University Hospitals and Clinics, Case Western Reserve University, Cleveland, OH 44106, USA

Bonnie J. Wakefield, PhD, RN
Research Scientist, Program for Interdisciplinary Research in Healthcare Organizations, Associate Chief Nursing Research, VA Medical Center, Iowa City, IA 52246, USA

Section I
Collaborative Healthware

I
Introduction: Care at a Distance

C. SAFRAN

The past three decades have seen revolutionary changes in health care but only evolutionary changes in healthcare information systems. This must change if we are to realize the full potential of collaborative care and shared decision making. Providers, patients, their families, and even payers must leverage the power of information technology to improve clinical care as well as satisfaction with that care, and to reduce costs.

Managed care and disease management have reduced the costs of care and excessive use of services, but compromised the physician's role and the patient's trust. With increasingly narrow profit margins for episodic care, or with outright capitated reimbursement models, health managers have sought to cut costs while increasing the number of encounters for which each physician is responsible. As the volume of care increases, clinicians must make sacrifices to spend more time with each patient. In fact, whereas the average duration of an ambulatory visit with a physician in the United States was 26 minutes in 1993, the current goal among health maintenance organizations is a 7-minute encounter (as in Great Britain).[1] A 7-minute visit with an elderly patient barely allows enough time for the patient to undress and dress again. A 7-minute encounter is too short to allow the physician to establish rapport, take a medical history, conduct a physical examination, formulate a therapeutic or diagnostic plan, and exchange information about the patient's concerns and the physician's proposed actions.

Medication errors may also result. Tamblyn et al[2] showed that when visits were shorter than 13 minutes, physicians made more medication errors than they made with longer visits. No wonder clinicians neglect to ask about alcohol and drug use, safety in the home, safe sex practices, and the health of other household members. No wonder both patients and physicians are increasingly dissatisfied with this model of care.

Another problem is that our current encounter-based model of care is both physician-centered and facility-centered. A patient who has a health concern must schedule an appointment at a time convenient for the physician and at the physician's office, which may be some distance from the patient's home. If

3

it turns out that the visit was unnecessary, both the patient's time and the physician's time will have been wasted. Alternatively, if the patient does not make a necessary visit because of the hassles of traveling for a 7-minute encounter, the patient's health could be compromised. This episodic approach not only leads to fragmented care but poorly supports both primary and longitudinal care.

In times past, clinicians could talk with their patients and take a complete history. They could build the trusting relationship so important to the art of healing. Sometimes physicians and nurses would even visit the patient's home and experience the patient as a person. This type of interaction is almost unthinkable in today's time-starved environment. But perhaps paradoxically, recent developments in broadband telecommunication and information technology may help us rebuild our eroding relationships with our patients.

Three advances in technology now allow us to interact with our patients when their health concerns first arise, or visit with our patients in their homes. Moreover, we can use this technology to engage patients in gathering and sharing information in ways that were inconceivable just a few years ago. First, with fast computers and reliable, inexpensive storage systems, we can now store nearly complete patient information, including images, sounds, and videos. Second, with collections of computer programs sometimes referred to as "electronic patient records," we can obtain, organize, display, and securely distribute this health information. Third, and perhaps most important, with the astounding growth of the Internet, we can anticipate radical changes in our society and culture, especially in the delivery of health care.

Fast affordable computing is penetrating our culture. Only 30 years ago, when I was in high school, the arrival of a single computer was a ribbon-cutting event. Today, an elementary school with no computer is considered disadvantaged. Only 20 years ago, when I finished my residency training, a disk drive that could store 200 million characters of text (about 70,000 typed pages) was the size of a washing machine and cost nearly $20,000.[3] Today a disk drive that holds several billion characters (one million typed pages) costs only $200 and will fit in a laptop computer. Within a few years, it will be possible to store trillions of characters on "smart cards" that patients could carry in their wallets. All the health data that are now collected could be stored indefinitely in central (or distributed) repositories and shared when appropriate.

But having large amounts of data and information will not be a panacea for clinicians or patients, since physicians do not have time to look through huge quantities of disorganized documents every time they need an item of data. The way clinical information is organized is equally important, and during the past 20 years, sophisticated software has been developed to support the flow of work in health care. Whether the enterprise is a large medical center[4,5] or a physician's office,[6,7] computer programs can collect patient information as a by-product of good patient care. Weed's[8] work on organizing clinical documents around the patient's problems not only led to the modern paper medical record but also influenced the development of such computing systems. To-day, the collection of programs that obtain patient information, display this information for the physician, and support the work flow is loosely referred to as the electronic patient record (a term that is misused by the nearly 400 com-panies that claim they can sell such a record and is misunderstood by most organizations that would like to buy one). Still, the ability to provide secure electronic access to patient information is a cornerstone to creative thinking about how we might reorganize the delivery of health care.

These improvements in computers and their applications have been dwarfed by the effects of the World Wide Web. The Internet itself is not new; in 1973 we could send electronic mail between university computers around the coun-try, exchange files including images, and even run computer programs remotely. What is new is the emergence of a common and intuitive interface that is accessible even to untrained users. In fact, the rate at which the World Wide Web has grown far exceeds the rate of growth of any other automated means of communication, including the telephone, the radio, and television.

As Internet traffic doubles every 5 months, with a yearly growth rate ex-ceeding 118%, we are seeing the emergence of the "wired health consumer," who has a computer at home and at work or school. We are seeing the telecom-munications and entertainment industry responding to pressure to sell inter-active video for use at home. What this means to health care is that our patients are already or will soon be online. In fact, of the 75 million free Internet searches of the MEDLINE database in 1997, 30% were conducted by the general public.[9]

How can more complex technology improve the healthcare environment I have described? Why would adding electronic tasks, such as answering e-mail from a patient, engaging in a virtual home visit via videoconferencing, updat-ing an electronic patient record, or even typing a prescription instead of illeg-ibly scribbling a script, help the time-hassled physician with only 7 minutes to see a patient? The reason is that with the more cooperative physician-patient relationship (and enhanced efficiency) the new technology allows, the patient can help with the routine collection and updating of health information.[10] In-formed and empowered, patients will communicate with their care team when a health concern arises. Perhaps the sight and sounds of the patient will trigger concerns that have the patient immediately come to the office or emergency room. Alternatively, computer-assisted histories will start a process of infor-mation exchange and shared decision making between the physician and pa-tient that could lead to diagnostic and therapeutic interventions before (or even without) an actual visit. Computer-assisted histories ask questions with-out observer bias and always ask every question that they are programmed to ask. Our experience with computer-assisted histories is that patients enjoy a well-constructed interview. The report of the computer interview saves time by highlighting important issues and sharing a documentation burden with the patient. The fear that physicians so often express that their patients will tell them too much is neither well founded in experience nor appropriate. Imagine that when asked by a computer (as should be done by every primary care doctor), "Are you depressed?" or "Do you have thoughts about hurting your-self?" doctors complain that they didn't want to know that information. Is there any excuse why we underdiagnose and treat depression other than we don't have enough time in a 7-minute visit to explore all these issues? The World Wide Web now gives us a means to have patients take a complete history before every visit. Even patients with poor eyesight with limited read-ing ability can respond to spoken questions that are easily incorporated within a Web interview.

Frequently, issues of equity arise when we consider extending care through the use of advanced home-based technology. While these concerns are appro-priate and real, work by Gustafson's group[11] and others suggests that this kind of technology has its greatest benefit for those populations of patients with the poorest access to care. Traditionally, we have thought about telemedicine (care at a distance) as providing access to care for patients who are at great distances from hospitals such as in rural settings. But within our urban centers where the majority of people live, many of the frail elderly and disenfranchised citizens will have the greatest health benefits from the application described in the following chapters.

The four chapters in this section demonstrate the next stage of collabora-tion in health care where cooperation among customers (individuals, families, and communities), suppliers (pharmaceutical, device manufacturers, and medi-cal supply companies), partners (national health systems, insurance compa-nies, and payers), and colleagues (physicians, nurses, other care providers, and support personnel) lets health systems do business in different and better ways. Since effective health care requires communication, consultation, and collaboration among colleagues as well as with patients, their families, and community resources, shouldn't healthcare information systems facilitate these basic tasks?

Clinicians need to embrace virtual patient visits as a way to revitalize our deteriorating relationship with our patients. We need to design this technol-ogy around the kind of care we seek to provide rather than responding piece-meal to administrative burdens. While adding more sophisticated technology to broken social systems almost never solves the human problem, sometimes high tech can also produce high touch. The following chapters show us how.

References

1. Davidoff F. Time. Ann Intern Med 1998.
2. Tamblyn R, Berkson, L, Dauphinee WD, et al. Unnecessary prescribing of NSAIDs and the management of NSAID-related gastropathy in medial practice. Ann Intern Med 1997;127:429–38.
3. Slack WV. Magnetic disk technology. MD Comput 1992;9:74–75.
4. Pryor TA, Gardner RM, Clayton PD, Warner HR. The HELP system. J Med Syst 1983;7:87–102.
5. Bleich HL, Beckley RF, Horowitz G, et al. Clinical computing in a teaching hospital. N Engl J Med 1985;312:756–764.

6. McDonald CJ. Tierney WM. Computer-stored medical records: their future role in medical practice. JAMA 1988;259:3433–3440.
7. Barnett GO. The application of computer-based medical record systems in ambulatory practice. N Engl J Med 1984;310:1645–1649.
8. Weed LL. Medical records that guide and teach. N Engl J Med 1968;278:593–600.
9. Lindberg DAB, Humphreys BL. Medicine and health on the Internet: the Good, the bad, and the ugly. JAMA 1998;280:1303–1304.
10. Safran C, Jones PC, Rind D, Bush B, Cytryn KN, Patel VL. Electronic communication and collaboration in a health care practice. Artif Intell Med 1998;12(2):139–153.
11. Pingree S, Hawkins RP, Gustafson DH, et al. Will the disadvantaged ride the information highway? J Broadcasting Electronic Media 1996;40:331–353.

1
Collaborative Healthware

D. Goldsmith and C. Safran

Patients are demanding a more substantive, collaborative role in their own healthcare decision making. Collaborative healthware is the application of information and communication technologies designed to enhance decision making and communication between providers, patients, and their families. The emergence of collaborative healthware will play an important role in supporting the relationship between patient and provider and will assist patients in better understanding their illness experience and how their own values affect decision making. Collaborative healthware is defined as "software for healthcare, tightly integrated with people systems"[1] and its creative and successful implementation will improve patient care and care management.

Collaborative healthware supports the relationship between healthcare provider and patient by engaging patients and their families as full partners in the healthcare process. In a collaborative partnership, patients expect that their clinicians will provide information and guidance. Patients expect that their clinicians will educate them and their families on illnesses, available therapies, potential outcomes, and complications, so that decisions can be made based on the patient's individual preferences.[2-5]

More often patients are presented with opportunities to actively participate in decisions that affect their lives and well-being.[6-9] While patient preferences for participation in clinical decisions vary greatly,[5,10,11] the desire for information about their health and health care is high.[12] Patients want information that addresses their individual concerns and conditions as well as interactive tools to manage their health and disease.[13,14] Providing patients with enhanced health-related information favorably affects their trust in, relationship with, and confidence in their healthcare providers.[15]

The actively engaged patient brings high expectations into healthcare relationships. These expectations can improve the way the system interacts with the patient and the way care is delivered.[4,7,16,17] Collaborative healthware enables patients to remold the more traditional physician-patient relationship to a more patient-centered relationship. To be effective partners in the management of their personal health, patients need information and education, as well as access and emotional support from their providers and care managers. To be effective and efficient in this partnership, providers and care managers need support from robust systems. Collaborative healthware provides the basic structure to advance this successful partnership.

Collaborative healthware solutions allow the development of prescribed healthcare communities that facilitate effective connectivity among participants. These solutions provide better access to information for patients, better distribution of expertise throughout the healthcare system, improved collaboration and coordination of care, and improved quality of care. The enabling technologies of collaborative healthware solutions are based on secure sharing of information and knowledge in a cost-effective manner.

Many of these systems described in the literature have been designed to support healthcare relationships and have been shown to improve clinical outcomes, reduce unnecessary service utilization, and generally increase satisfaction.[4,18-23] Participants in these communities may include patients, family members, physicians, other members of the clinical team, health plan case managers, nurse advisors, and employers, among others.

Studies have shown that interactive health communication (IHC) systems such as CHESS have the potential to enhance health, minimize burden of illness, and optimize relationships between consumers and their health providers.[24] CHESS has been shown to be well used and well liked by patients.[8,25] While the emphasis of IHC is on the interaction of the individual with technology, the emphasis of collaborative healthware is on the collaboration between two or more stakeholders. Collaborative healthware builds on the value of IHC in that it provides a technical structure that facilitates a partnership between patient and provider where knowledge transfer and shared decision making is the expectation.

The informed and actively engaged patient is more likely to comply with therapy, proactively report new or changing symptoms, and see himself as a partner in the care process.[26] The processes underlying the creation and maintenance of healthcare relationships are complex, ill-defined, and executed with varying degrees of success. Ultimately, any breaks in this complex system of delivering care manifest themselves in both additional costs and decreased patient satisfaction.

Technology can play an important role in restoring relationships between patients and the healthcare system. Technology can facilitate improvement in quality, cost, and patient satisfaction. Properly applied Internet technology can be used successfully as a platform on which to deliver interventions to patients that significantly enhance the outcomes of care.[19]

A Framework for Patient–Provider Collaboration

Supporting patient–provider collaboration with technology requires an underlying framework to facilitate participation. Goldberg et al[26,27] suggest a framework for patient empowerment and the technical realization of that framework. Such a framework is a requirement for properly designed collaborative healthware applications. This framework consists of core elements essential to facilitating patients' active participation in their own health care: targeted and personalized patient education, access to personally relevant credible information, ongoing and facilitated communication, clinical data capture, a reporting and feedback mechanism, and community support. In addition to this framework, other issues must be considered prior to the design, implementation, and evaluation of collaborative healthware.[13] Such consideration should include:

- What do patients need?
- What do providers want?
- How can the patients' "view" be designed into the system?
- How can prescribed, profile-driven knowledge be delivered?
- What are the best methods of information delivery?
- How can credible data be collected from patients?
- How can the system be integrated into the current work flow?

The Digital Divide

Unfortunately, there has always been a gap between those people and communities who have access to the newest technology available and those who do not. The term *digital divide* is used to refer to this gap. While there are conflicting reports on the extent of the divide, most agree that a divide does exist. *A Nation Online: How Americans Are Expanding Their Use of the Internet*[28] reports on the rapidly growing use of new information technologies such as the Internet across all demographic groups and geographic regions.

More than half of the nation (54%) is now online and the rate of growth of Internet use in the United States is currently two million new Internet users per month. The profile of computer and Internet users demonstrates that the rise in computer and Internet use is spread across a wide range of the population. Internet use is increasing for people regardless of income, education, age, race, ethnicity, or gender.[28]

While Internet use continues to rise among people who live in lower income households, family income remains the main indicator of whether a person is likely to use a computer or the Internet. Individuals who live in high-income households are more likely to be computer and Internet users than those who live in low-income households.[28] Internet use has also increased across all races and groups. White Americans continue to be the largest segment of the population using computers despite the fact that growth rates in Internet use were faster for blacks and Hispanics. Between August 2000 and September 2001, Internet use among blacks and Hispanics increased at annual rates of 33% and 30%, respectively. Whites, Asian Americans, and Pacific Islanders experienced annual growth rates of approximately 20% during these same periods.[28]

In addition to family income and race, educational attainment also factors into computer and Internet use. The higher a person's level of education, the more likely he or she will be a computer or Internet user. Adults with education beyond college were the most likely to be both computer and Internet users. Adults whose highest level of education is less than high school were less likely to be both computer and Internet users. Encouraging trends indicate that Internet use is growing rapidly among those with lower levels of educational attainment.[28]

Manhattan Research data show that in 2002 some 63 million Americans were e-health consumers.[29] Unfortunately, health literacy and reading level are both significant contributors to the digital divide.[30] Low health literacy can have an impact on anyone regardless of age, race, education, or income level. Patients who have difficulty understanding the health information they are provided with are at higher risk for poor health outcomes.

Current efforts to lessen the digital divide have focused on providing ubiquitous access to computers and the Internet. The establishment of community computer/Internet centers in low-income neighborhoods has been supported by various foundations, corporations, local businesses, and government agencies. Many federal departments financially support programs that promote access to computers, the Internet, telemedicine, and reliable health information.[31] Several national health objectives look to expand access to the Internet at home, improve health literacy, and improve the quality of online resources.[32] More recently, attention is being directed at the development of software applications designed specifically for the economically disadvantaged.

Economically Disadvantaged Families with Premature Infants

For families that depend on Medicaid support, the emotional, social, and economic toll of serious illness is magnified not only by circumstance, but also by stereotyped preconception. For instance, Medicaid mothers who have preterm infants in neonatal intensive care units (NICUs) are younger, have attained lower levels of education, may have had less prenatal care, and have more children at home than do mothers who have paid for in vitro fertilization. However, the circumstance of being poor and receiving support from Medicaid does not imply that a parent lacks the motivation or intelligence to use e-health applications. On the contrary, a mother of a sick child is a powerful advocate for her child's health regardless of socioeconomic status. Collaborative healthware can be a valuable and effective approach for this medically underserved and disadvantaged population that makes up such a large proportion of those families with low birth weight or medically complex newborns requiring NICU care.

Many medically fragile infants have complex chronic medical problems that place them at higher risk for postdischarge mortality, childhood morbidity from acute and chronic illnesses, and long-term developmental/ educational difficulties. Those infants who are born into socioeconomically disadvantaged families are faced with even greater risk because they lack the financial resources and adequate social and emotional support they need. Providing Medicaid parents with the resources of collaborative healthware will enhance the early identification of critical issues facing families prior to and upon integration into the community with a medically complex infant.

The admission of a baby into an NICU is one of the most challenging and distressing episodes in the lives of parents as they grieve the loss of a normal pregnancy, are overwhelmed by the foreign and distressing NICU environment, experience a roller coaster of emotions, and are often cut off from their usual support structures. During this most difficult time, collaborative healthware applications can be used to encourage a sense of control as parents receive daily updates and pictures of their infant. These applications can also enhance parent-NICU communication with secure messaging capabilities and improve knowledge transfer though personalized discharge teaching modules. Following discharge, families must cope with the transition from the highly monitored NICU environment to the less intense, but perhaps more intimidating, situation of having a high-risk infant at home.

Despite the fact that compliance with postdischarge programs may help prevent adverse outcomes for their infant, many Medicaid families have a hard time following up with recommended medical care and developmental services. Collaborative healthware applications can be used to support care coordination and follow-up monitoring and facilitate ongoing communication with parents and care partners. Early identification of issues facing families upon integration into the community avoids costly readmissions and helps to decrease the stress associated with caring for a premature or low birth weight newborn.

Collaborative healthware applications offer a comprehensive, organized platform for families to document issues for discussion with their primary physician, track their infant's progress toward developmental milestones, and maintain accurate, up-to-date immunization records. Parents can access a knowledge base particular to infants who experienced an NICU stay and who may have ongoing medical problems and/or an anticipated developmental timeline that differs from that expected with a full-term healthy infant. Early recognition by parents of a delay in reaching critical milestones helps ensure that an infant's potential is maximized. In addition, parents are provided with the early warning signs that their baby may need to be seen by a physician. This helps parents identify potentially serious clinical problems before they progress and lead to emergency care and/or rehospitalization. This information can be delivered at predetermined intervals such as during flu and allergy seasons to serve as a reminder. Collaborative healthware applications can make the challenges associated with taking a baby home from the NICU a bit easier for parents and for the clinicians who care for them.

Baby CareLink

Mount Sinai Medical Center (MSMC), in partnership with the State of Illinois Department of Public Aid, is using collaborative healthware in their NICU to support Medicaid parents with low birth weight and medically complex newborns. MSMC has implemented CST Baby CareLink, in both English and Spanish, to improve communication, increase family participation, enhance parent education, and facilitate more effective discharge planning. A pilot study implementation of this e-health initiative has resulted in improved parent engagement, decreased length of stay, a low readmission rate, and high NICU nurse satisfaction.

Using the collaborative healthware Baby CareLink system, parents can receive daily updates from the NICU, track information about their baby's health, see recent pictures of their baby, communicate with NICU staff, access a personalized knowledge base for newborn care, and provide feedback regarding the care process. Using Baby CareLink, NICU nurses can communicate with families, personalize discharge planning and baby care education, and access a medical reference library. Following discharge, Baby CareLink can be used to support care coordination, follow-up monitoring, and ongoing communication with parents, with the goal of reducing emergency department visits or rehospitalization.

After 9 months of use at MSMC, an initial evaluation was completed. During this period, 228 infants supported by Medicaid were enrolled into Baby CareLink. Eighty-one percent of the enrolled parents spoke English, and 19% spoke Spanish. Average length of stay in the NICU for infants whose families were using Baby CareLink was 2.73 days less than for those at Mount Sinai during the same period 1 year earlier, before Baby CareLink was installed. Follow-up information for babies enrolled in the pilot and born more than 6 months prior to the evaluation revealed that only three of 17 infants (18%) experienced a readmission during the period; this is far less than the expected 40% readmission rate for this population. This decrease in average length of stay and low readmission rate yields significant medical cost savings.

Along with cost savings, medical staff also reported very high satisfaction with Baby CareLink as a care support tool. Nursing staff members who were surveyed 6 months after Baby CareLink was installed in the unit reported that Baby CareLink improved NICU nursing staff communication with families; increased family members' comfort, confidence, and competency in caring for their infant; increased parent participation with nurses and their infants during the NICU stay; and overall helped the nurse and the family. Nursing staff also reported that parents using Baby CareLink visited the NICU more frequently while their infants were admitted.

During the evaluation period, there were 2349 log-ins to Baby CareLink. Sixty-four percent of parents accessed Baby CareLink from computer terminals installed specifically for their use in the MSMC NICU, and 36% accessed Baby

CareLink from home, school, library, or their workplace. Many of the young parents who were still in high school accessed Baby CareLink from the school library during their lunch breaks. Either way, parents were reading the assigned educational material designed to help them better understand the medical condition of their infant and help prepare them for their infants' discharge to home. The type of material accessed most often by parents included preparing for discharge (17%), welcome and home page information (15%), getting to know and see your baby (14%), and daily report and other clinical information (13%).

Parental discharge teaching, which was previously concentrated on the day of discharge, is now initiated earlier and provided over a more extended period of time using Baby CareLink. Parents are more motivated to learn and prefer the autonomy and ability to control the pace of their learning using the computer system on their own. Clinicians review with the parents any questions they have after reading the assigned Baby CareLink learning modules and assess their comprehension of the material. As a result of the targeted, personalized education, parents ask more informed questions and understand their challenges much better. Clinicians believe that parents who use Baby CareLink are more confident about caring for their children and are prepared to take the infants home sooner.

Collaborative healthware has been integrated into the normal operation of the Mount Sinai NICU, and Web site usage data suggest that Medicaid parents are successfully using the application. Early evidence from the parents, nurses, social workers, and doctors indicates a positive impact on the parents' competence and confidence in caring for their fragile infants. How successfully it will be used by Medicaid families in the community following the infant's discharge from the NICU and whether it produces health/cost-effective results is currently under review.

The Pediatric Oncology Population

Acute lymphoblastic leukemia (ALL) accounts for about 80% of the childhood cases of leukemia in the United States; approximately 3000 new cases of ALL are diagnosed in the United States each year.[33] The development of effective therapy for children with ALL is one of the undisputed successes of modern clinical hematology-oncology. Fifty years ago ALL was uniformly fatal, but currently over three quarters of children with ALL are cured.[34] Improvement in outcomes over the last 40 years can be attributed to the development of complex chemotherapeutic regimens.

Patients with ALL generally receive treatment for 2 to 3 years, a significant portion of which is now given while the patient resides at home. Parents who participate in home chemotherapy report that administering the chemotherapy treatments themselves helped them to cope with the disease, feel more in control, and learn more about their child's illness and treatment.[35] However, the proper administration of these potentially lifesaving medications in the home is a safety issue. Patients and families must learn to manage medications, mitigate side effects, and watch for potential complications while adhering to treatment protocol. A number of high-risk events are commonly associated with this form of therapy, including leukopenia, bleeding diathesis, and opportunistic infections. The parent is responsible to monitor the child for compliance with the oral chemotherapy agents and for side effects of the treatment regimen, including infection and complications with venous catheters. Close monitoring and follow-up with the healthcare team are required for many years.[36,37]

Parents' information needs during home chemotherapy include the details of managing daily care tasks, conceptual information about disease and treatment, and sources of emotional and psychological support. Parents generally prefer to get information about their child's illness from the medical staff; however, clinicians may have limited time to teach parents during the medical encounter. Under stress, parents may have limited ability to absorb what they are told. Parents of children with ALL are struggling to manage the complexity of their child's care in the home.[14] These parents have been creative in finding ways to adapt and cope with the challenges that face them, but they have an urgent need for tools that will help them to organize the care needs of their child as well as to recognize early the appearance of medication side effects.

Computers are an increasing source of health-related information, but the questions and concerns of family caregivers almost always go beyond the generally available patient education information on the Internet. In a study of the information-seeking behavior of parents of children with ALL, the most frequent parent queries concerned practical issues such as current blood counts, indications of the progress of the disease, the vulnerability of the child to infection, whether something would make the child sick, and what should be done about fever and vomiting.[38] Parents require up-to-date, personally relevant, and easily accessible information. Parents in one study agreed that having relevant health information on their child's own personal health Web site, to be available to them at the time when they were ready to hear it and when they most needed it, would be highly beneficial to the care of their child with ALL.[14] This is consistent with previous work, which demonstrated that Web-based education used by patients at a time that was most convenient and relevant to them would in fact improve their clinical outcomes.[6,18-20]

Internet-based collaborative healthware applications designed to support the home management of childhood leukemia connects the family and patient in the home with their care team at the cancer center. These applications incorporate innovative care support tools that families of children with ALL can use in their homes to help them manage medications, side effects of treatment, and potential complications. Access to protocol-driven, personalized medication schedules, a medication administration record, and decision support tools that recognize and report medication side effects assists the care team in recognizing urgent or life-threatening situations. Experience to date suggests that parents of children with ALL consider care support tools such as these highly beneficial and would use them if they were shown to improve the care of their child.[14]

Conclusion

Experience with collaborative healthware applications in vulnerable populations suggests that families from all walks of life will use and benefit from collaborative tools that keep them informed and involved in the care of their children. While access to computer hardware and the Internet continue to be barriers to the implementation of such applications, the most significant barrier continues to be the lack of applications designed specifically for those with the greatest need. Several national health objectives are expanding access to the Internet and to quality online resources for disadvantaged populations, which is an important first step. Innovative design and implementation of collaborative healthware applications, however, have the potential to improve the health care of these populations through better collaboration and communication.

With widespread adoption of collaborative healthware applications, all patients and their families will come to expect improved access to services, greater convenience, and alternative methods of communicating with their healthcare providers. Since the emphasis is on the partnership between patient and provider, collaborative healthware will be used to promote informed decision making, improve patient outcomes, increase patient satisfaction, enhance patient education, lower healthcare costs, and improve the coordination of care. While collaborative healthware applications have intuitive appeal to diverse groups of healthcare stakeholders, adoption of such systems will likely depend on their ability to demonstrate positive impact on outcomes.

References

1. Safran C. The collaborative edge: patient empowerment for vulnerable populations. Int J Med Informatics 2002;1–6.
2. Ferguson T. Consumer health informatics. HealthCare Forum 1995;28–33.
3. Mandl KD, Kohane IS, Brandt AM. Electronic patient-physician communication: problems and promise. Ann Intern Med 1998;129(6):495–500.
4. Slack VW. Cybermedicine: how computing empowers patients for better healthcare. Medinfo 1998;1:3–5.
5. Brennan PF. Health informatics and community health: support for patients as collaborators in care. Methods Inform Med 1999;38(4-5):274–278.
6. Brennan PF, Ripich S. Use of a home care computer network by persons with AIDS. Int J Technol Assess Health Care 1994;10(2):258–272.
7. Ferguson T. Online patient-helpers and physicians working together: a new patient

collaboration for high quality health care. BMJ 2000;321(7269):1129–1132.

8. Gustafson DH, Hawkins RP, Boberg EW, et al. CHESS: ten years of research and development in consumer health informatics for broad populations, including the underserved. Medinfo 2001;10(2):14590–1563.

9. Porter SC. Patients as experts: a collaborative performance support system. Proc AMIA Symposium 2001;548–552.

10. Benbassat J, Pilpel D, Tidhar M. Patients' preferences for participation in clinical decision making: a review of published surveys. Behav Med 1998;24(2):81–88.

11. Brennan PF, Strombom I. Improving health care by understanding patient preferences: the role of computer technology. JAMIA 1998;5(3):257–262.

12. Tang PC, Newcomb C, Gorden S, Kreider N. Meeting the information needs of patients: results from a patient focus group. Proc AMIA Annual Fall Symposium 1997;672–676.

13. Kaplan B, Brennan PF. Consumer informatics: supporting patients as co-producers of quality. JAMIA 2001;8(4):309–316.

14. Goldsmith D, Silverman LB, Safran C. (2002). Pediatric Cancer CareLink: supporting home management of childhood leukemia. Proc AMIA Symposium 2002;290–294.

15. Tang PC, Newcomb C. Informing patients: a guide for providing patient health information. JAMIA 1998;5(6):563–570.

16. Slack VW, Slack CW. Patient computer dialog. N Engl J Med 1972;286(24):1304–1309.

17. Landro L. Patient-physician communication: an emerging partnership. Oncologist 1999;4(1):55–58.

18. Brennan PF. Characterizing the use of health care services delivered via computer networks. JAMIA 1995;2(3):160–168.

19. Goldsmith D, Safran C. Using the web to reduce postoperative pain following ambulatory surgery. Proc AMIA Symposium 1999;6:780–784.

20. Gray J, Safran C, Weitzner GP, Steward JE, Zaccagnini L, Pursley D. Baby CareLink: using the Internet and telemedicine to improve care for high-risk infants. Pediatrics 2000;106:1318–1324.

21. Gustafson DH, McTavish F, Hawkins RP, et al. Computer support for elderly women with breast cancer. JAMA 1998;280(15):1305.

22. Safran C, Jones PC, Rind D, Bush B, Cytryn KN, Patel VL. Electronic communication and collaboration in a health care practice. Artif Intell Med 1998;12(2):139–153.

23. Vandenberg TA, Gustafson DH, Owen B, et al. Interaction between the breast cancer patient and the health care system. Cancer Prevent Control 1997;1(2):152–153.

24. Eng T, Gustafson D, eds. Wired for health and well being: the emergence of interactive health communication. Washington, DC: U.S. Department of Health and Human Services, 1999.

25. Gustafson DH, McTavish F, Boberg E, et al. Empowering patients using computer based health support systems. Qual Health Care 1999;8(1):49–56.

26. Goldberg HS, Safran C. Support for the cancer patient: an Internet model. In: Silva J, Ball MJ, Chute CG, et al., eds. Cancer informatics: essential technologies for clinical trials. New York: Springer-Verlag, 2002:280–292.

27. Goldberg HS, Morales A, Gottlieb L, Meador L, Safran C. Reinventing patient

centered computing for the twenty-first century. In: Patel V, et al., eds. MedInfo 2001. Amsterdam: IOS Press, 2001:1455–1458.

28. U.S. Department of Commerce. A nation online: how Americans are expanding their use of the Internet. http://www.ntia.doc.gov/ntiahome/dn, 2002.

29. Manhattan Research. For 124.7 million Americans, the Internet is no longer considered "alternative medicine." October 17, 2002 news release. http://www.manhattanresearch.com/inthenews.htm, 2002.

30. Eng TR, Maxfield A, Patrick K, Deering MJ, Ratzan S, Gustafson D. Access to health information and support: a public highway or a private road? JAMA 1998;280:1371–1375.

31. U.S. Department of Health and Human Services. Information for health: a strategy for building the National Health Information Infrastructure. Washington, DC: U.S. Government Printing Office, 2001.

32. Healthy People 2010. U.S. Department of Health and Human Services, Office of Disease Prevention and Health Promotion. http://www.hhs.gov; http://odphp.osophs.dhhs.gov; http://nnlm.gov/partners/hp/.

33. Ries LAG, Smith MA, Gurney JG, et al. Cancer incidence and survival among children and adolescents: United States SEER Program 1975-1995. NIH publication No. 99-4649. Bethesda, MD: National Cancer Institute, 1999.

34. Silverman LB, Gelber RD, Dalton VK, et al. Improved outcome for children with acute lymphoblastic leukemia: results of Dana-Farber Consortium Protocol 91-01. Blood 2001;97:1211.

35. Hooker L, Kohler J. Safety, efficacy, and acceptability of home intravenous therapy administered by parents of pediatric oncology patients. Med Pediatr Oncol 1999;32(6):421–462.

36. Close P, Burkey E, Kazak A, Lange B. (1995). A prospective, controlled evaluation of home chemotherapy for children with cancer. Pediatrics, 1995;95(6):896–9003.

37. Davies HA, Lilleyman JS. Compliance with oral chemotherapy in childhood lymphoblastic leukaemia. Cancer Treat Rev 1995;21(2):93–103.

38. Tetzlaff L. Consumer informatics in chronic illness. JAMIA 1997;4(4):285–3006.

2
PatientSite: Patient-Centered Communication, Services, and Access to Information

DANIEL Z. SANDS AND JOHN D. HALAMKA

Healthcare providers are not meeting the needs of online consumers. Over half the U.S. population is currently online and the place they turn for health information, after their doctors, is the Internet[1] (Fig. 2.1). In another survey, Internet users were almost as likely to turn to the Internet for healthcare information as they were their physician.[2]

Although 45% of online consumers would like to communicate with their physicians using e-mail, only 6% have done so.[1] Similar proportions of people have and would like to access a provider Web site (Fig. 2.2). Moreover, almost half of consumers who would like to do so would be willing to switch providers to find one who offered these services.[1] The proportion of those who have gone online to look for health information is 66% to 78% of those who have used the Internet, and that number is growing annually.[2,3]

Online health consumers want the same kind of convenience they expect from other businesses today. They want to be able to communicate by e-mail, get information, and conduct transactions conveniently. In surveys, consumers consistently tell us the types of things they would like to do online: consult with their physicians about medical issues, refill their prescriptions, make appointments, look up their test results, and find information about health problems.[1,4]

Healthcare Consumer Needs

Communication

Although there are many channels available for patient-provider communication, including in-person interaction, telephone, fax, and page, patient-provider interactions are generally restricted to appointments and telephone calls. Because both of these are synchronous communication channels, busy patients and overbooked providers have difficulty making contact. As most of the world gravitates toward asynchronous electronic communication for nonurgent communication, it seems clear that electronic patient-centered com-

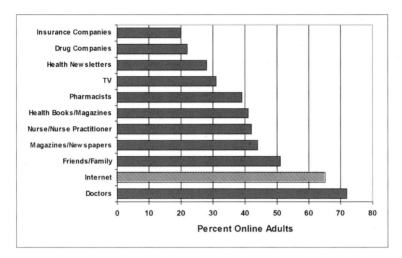

FIGURE 2.1. Sources consumers use for health information. (From Manhattan Research, LLC. Reprinted with permission.)

munication such as e-mail would be useful in patient-provider interactions. Unfortunately, although half the U.S. population uses e-mail, only about 25% of physicians have used e-mail to communicate with their patients[5] and probably only 10% to 15% use it regularly.

E-mail has a number of beneficial characteristics when used according to a set of guidelines.[6] The asynchronous nature of e-mail allows users to send and read message at their convenience. Unlike telephone calls, which courtesy dictates cannot be used outside of certain hours, one may communicate electronically any time of the day or night. Also, instead of a rushed telephone

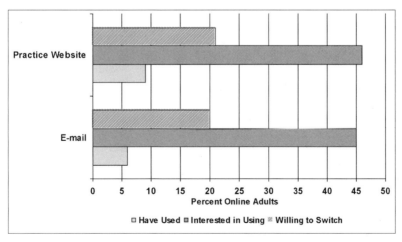

FIGURE 2.2. Consumer demand for practice Web site and physician e-mail. (From Manhattan Research, LLC. Reprinted with permission.)

conversation or brief appointment, patients may take their time composing their questions, and physicians can do research before responding. In addition, unlike telephone conversations, which are often not documented adequately in the patient record, e-mail is self-documenting, providing a convenient transcript of the interaction that can be filed in the patient's record. This also permits patients to reflect on their providers' comments and discuss them with friends and family members. In contrast to an appointment, e-mail communication is informal, most akin to a telephone call. Using e-mail improves communication between patients and their providers and increases patient satisfaction.

However, e-mail has some drawbacks when used for electronic patient-centered communication. For one thing, because e-mail has no linkage to the record of the patient with whom the discussion is taking place, it is both cumbersome to archive and difficult to determine the context of a patient's question (one must correctly determine the patient's identity and pull the record). Another issue is that messages are typically unstructured, and this may reduce the efficiency of communication. Also, in many practices, patients can send e-mail only to their physician rather than to other persons in the practice. This means that the physician must triage all incoming messages himself and deliver them to the appropriate person(s) in the practice. Finally, e-mail as generally used is an insecure channel of communication; messages can be read inadvertently or intentionally by third parties. It is this last issue that some fear may make clinical use of unencrypted e-mail a violation of the Health Insurance Portability and Accountability Act (HIPAA).

Information

It is clear that patients who use the Internet want access to health information. For most of the history of medicine, health information has been the exclusive province of the medical practitioner. This information asymmetry, where the physician knows everything and the patient knows nothing, has been a source of comfort to physicians, but is contradictory to the free flow of information that the Internet has brought about. Health information is available through tens of thousands of Web sites, many of which have reliable information. Patients want to learn about health promotion, medical conditions, and treatments.[1]

Patient also want access to their medical records, medications, allergies, problem lists, appointment history, and even their test results. HIPAA requires that we let patients view their medical records, but it's still a quite cumbersome process in most institutions. If patients have better access to information, they can be more active participants in their health.

Convenience

Most people who use the Web are accustomed to online "convenience" transactions, such as ordering airline tickets, contacting customer support, and ordering or returning merchandise. In health care, we offer almost none of these conveniences to our customers. Patients who need prescription refills, appointments, managed care referrals, or answers to a billing question, or who need to update their contact information must negotiate these tasks through telephone calls. This leads to patient frustration and inefficiency on both ends of the conversation. Clearly, we can offer better service, and patients have a right to expect these services to be available online.

By recognizing the needs of online healthcare consumers, healthcare institutions can work to meet them. In 1999 at CareGroup Healthcare System, we initiated a project to address these issues.

CareGroup and Beth Israel Deaconess Medical Center

CareGroup Healthcare System is an integrated healthcare delivery system based in Boston, Massachusetts. It comprises five hospitals (including the flagship, Beth Israel Deaconess Medical Center) and 1700 medical staff who provide care for more than one million patients through many affiliated practices. CareGroup has been at the forefront of technologic innovation in health care since it implemented one of the world's first clinical computing systems, the CCC system, a quarter-century ago,[7,8] and the online medical record in 1989.[9] The CCC system also contained one of the first e-mail systems to be used in a clinical facility. CareGroup was named the most technologically advanced healthcare company in America by Information Week magazine.

Beth Israel Deaconess Medical Center has a legacy of patient-centered care. In the 1970s we did trials of interviewing patients using computers[10] and early experiments of giving patients their medical records to bring to their appointments.[11] Beth Israel was also the home of one of the first divisions of academic general internal medicine.[12] In the 1980s the primary nursing movement and other nursing care innovations were implemented at Beth Israel.[13] Beth Israel Hospital began a program, funded by the Picker/Commonwealth Patient-Centered Care program, to survey patients about their healthcare experiences.[14] In the 1990s, we started a patient-family learning center[15] for patients, their caregivers, and the general public. One of the authors (D.Z.S.), who practices medicine at Beth Israel Deaconess Medical Center, had been actively promoting the use of e-mail in patient care through policy and educational efforts at the national level.

The PatientSite Project[16]

In 1999 members of the CareGroup information system (IS) and Beth Israel Deaconess Medical Center's Division of General Medicine began discussing how to best involve patients in their care and meet the needs of online patients. As elements of this, we wanted to allow patients to see their records online and communicate securely with their healthcare providers. We decided that the best way to do this was through a Web site using secure sockets layer (SSL) encryption.

To execute this, the group initially met with an outside company to do the programming, but we later realized that it would be more efficient to do the programming internally. We developed this using Microsoft Internet Information Server, Microsoft SQL database, and active server pages with server-side scripting to maintain client platform independence. Displaying the patient record information from the CCC system through a Web browser was done using technology developed by one of the authors (J.D.H.) in a project called CareWeb.[17]

In April 2000 we began registering physicians, staff, and patients in a single practice. We gradually added a small number of other CareGroup practices, physicians, and patients. By August 2000 we had more than 1000 patients online, as well as 43 physicians in 10 practices. We declared the pilot a success and moved to wider deployment. As of February 2003 we had 120 physicians in 40 practices using PatientSite and had enrolled 11,000 patients.

Design and Implementation Considerations

We wanted to build PatientSite using standard tools. This included the server software, programming language, database, and security tools. We wanted to strike a balance between usability and security, recognizing that a system that was too well protected would require trade-offs of usability. Physicians would need to endure an extra layer of security, however, because they would have access to personal information from all of their patients, whereas patients would have access only to information about themselves.

At the time we developed PatientSite, there were many types of Web browsers in common use, so we utilized mainly server-side scripting to maintain browser independence. This imposed serious limitations in our user interface design. Later, Microsoft's Internet Explorer became the most commonly used browser. We in turn conformed to the capabilities of Internet Explorer, which afforded us more flexibility in user interface design.

From an implementation standpoint, we wanted users to initiate the registration process online and then complete the process through a telephone interaction. We considered requiring personal contact to register patients, but so as not to impede the registration process, we discarded this in favor of allowing the confirmation to take place via telephone.

We wanted to enable physicians to control how PatientSite worked for them. For example, we felt that physicians should decide which features of PatientSite their patient could use and how their messages should be routed.

Security

PatientSite is a secure Web site that uses SSL with 128-bit encryption. Users access it by logging in with a user name and password. We considered some of the advanced security used in the Patient-Centered Access to Secure Systems Online (PCASSO) project,[18] but felt that a complicated multistep log-in procedure would be too cumbersome for wide deployment among physicians and patients. After all, many of these same patients had been using unencrypted e-mail to discuss medical issues; a password-protected secure Web site provided protection well beyond that. For physicians we did require a second layer of authentication, for which we initially used SecureID.[19] This was an expensive technology to use and support, however, and was prone to failure; two thirds of the log-in attempts were unsuccessful, and managing the hardware tokens proved problematic. We later settled on using physicians' clinical information system log-in IDs as the secondary authentication mechanism.

Secure Communication

One of the features of PatientSite is secure messaging. Users (patients, staff, and providers) have a mailbox on PatientSite that allows them to send messages to other users on PatientSite. No clinical information ever leaves the secure Web site. When a message arrives, recipients are alerted via an unencrypted e-mail message sent through regular e-mail. Recipients can then click on the PatientSite URL, their Web browser will open, and they can log in to read their message.

The functions of the PatientSite mailbox are in many ways similar to those of an ordinary e-mail program. Each message has a subject and a body. Messages can be composed, read, sent, and forwarded to others. Other features differ from e-mail. Each message has a classification, such as "clinical," "referral," and "prescription." Because messages have a classification, they can be automatically routed to those who can best handle them (e.g., prescription requests to the prescription staff). We allowed physicians to dictate routing of these various message types. By default, clinical messages would be handled directly by the physician.

Services for Patients

In addition to secure messaging, PatientSite allows patients to perform "convenience" transactions online. This includes requesting appointments, obtaining prescription renewals, requesting managed-care referrals, and viewing their bills.

Patients wishing to have a nonurgent appointment may (if their physician has permitted it) view the physicians schedule and fill out a Web-based form specifying when they would like the appointment. We considered permitting patients to actually book themselves into their physicians' schedules, but we felt that booking a medical appointment online is not the same, for example, as buying airline tickets online; it requires human intervention to make sure the scheduling is appropriate based on physician, patient, and scheduling factors. The appointment request is sent and reviewed by whomever the physician has designated as being responsible for managing these requests. The patient is

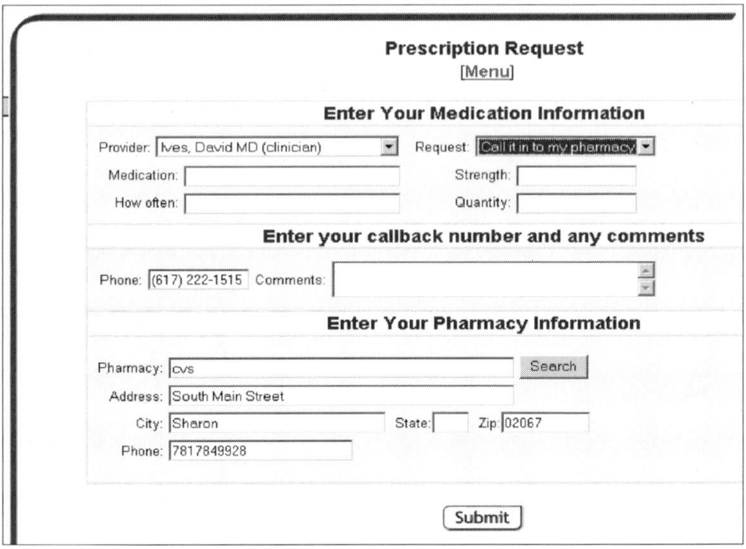

Figure 2.3. PatientSite prescription request.

contacted either through secure messaging or by telephone to complete the booking.

PatientSite similarly allows patients to request prescription renewals using online forms. In this case, the patient specifies not only details about the prescription but also delivery instructions for the prescription. Prescription information is automatically completed when the patient uses the refill button next to a medication on the medication list screen (Fig. 2.3). The prescription can be left for the patient to pick up, or the patient can specify that the prescription should be mailed to them or should be called in to a specific pharmacy. Each patient's favorite pharmacy is the default, but other pharmacy information may be entered; a pharmacy lookup is provided as a reference. In addition, when patients need specialty referrals, online referral forms enable them to request the referral from their primary care physician.

All of these requests generate a message on PatientSite. While many of them can be processed by support staff without physician involvement (if the physician has designated others in the office to handle them), the messages may be routed back to the physician if there are questions about them. Prescriptions sometimes require a physician's signature, as do managed-care referrals.

We also enable patients to view their bills online, something only possible if the patient's physician uses our centralized billing system.

Physicians can control both the handling of messages and whether to enable patients to request prescription refills, appointments, and managed-care referrals or to view their schedule.

Patient Education

Every patient's "home page" on PatientSite contains customizable health education links (Fig. 2.4). These may be "prescribed" or suggested to a patient by a physician through a message (often to support a response to the patient) or they may be selected directly by the patient. Discrete links may be added, but patients can also select predefined collections of links, clustered by category. These collections are managed by our patient education committee.

Patients may also view drug information monographs about each of their drugs by clicking on the drug of interest that appears on their medication list. In this way they can better understand their medications, how to take them, and what adverse effects can result.

Integration with Record

All patients registered on PatientSite have links to their records that are established at the time of registration. Once this is done, it is possible for patients to view their records online. Patients may see most aspects of their record online, including medication lists, problem lists, allergies, and all test results (except initial HIV test results). If the patient's physician does not use computerized patient records or does not have tests performed through one of our affiliated medical centers, these elements will not be viewable.

We wish to emulate best practice with respect to storing online communication. Therefore, clinicians can view all messages sent through PatientSite through a "Messages" section of the clinical information system. All PatientSite messages are archived as long as the rest of our clinical information.

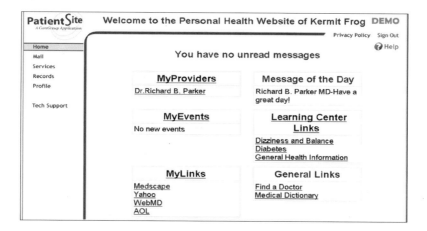

FIGURE 2.4. Patient home page on PatientSite showing health education links.

Personal Health Record

Patients can maintain their own record on PatientSite. They can record their own medications, problems, allergies, and notes. They can also track and graph data over time, such as blood glucose measurements, weights, blood pressure, symptom scores, and other quantitative information. Finally, they can upload files, including images, documents, and spreadsheets.

Results

Since the implementation of PatientSite in April 2000, we have monitored its use both by patients and providers. Figure 2.5 shows the enrollment over time of patients and physicians in PatientSite. We counted as active users only the patients who logged on and electronically signed the usage agreement after they were enrolled.

As of February 2003 PatientSite had 11,103 active patients, defined as patients who had logged on at least once after they had been registered. The median age was 43, with 4% over the age of 70; 57% were female.

The 121 attending physicians came from 40 different CareGroup practices. In addition to several primary care practices, PatientSite physicians came from a number of different specialty practices, including allergy, cardiology, hematology-oncology, nephrology, obstetrics-gynecology, and pulmonology. There are also 225 support staff registered on PatientSite, such as secretarial, nursing, and appointment staff.

As of this writing, we have begun to register nonphysician clinicians on PatientSite, including nurse-midwives and nurse practitioners. We are in the planning stages of enrolling residents.

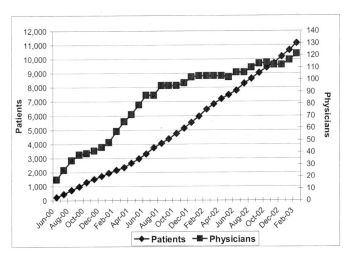

FIGURE 2.5. Active users of PatientSite.

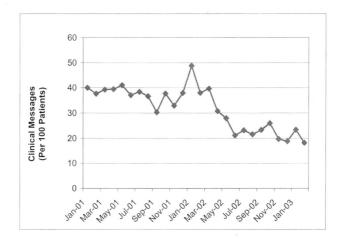

FIGURE 2.6. Clinical messages over time.

One of the ways to show a system is useful is to show that it is used over time by voluntary users[7, 8, 20, 21] We also wanted to begin to understand the work flow implications of this new communication medium. We therefore examined the volume of messages sent each month over time. We broke the messages down by type, since different messages are handled by different members of the practices. For example, clinical messages are almost always sent directly to physicians, while prescription requests are generally handled by nonphysician staff.

Since the message volume would be proportional to the volume of users, we adjusted the monthly message volume by dividing by the number of users and multiplying that by 100 to give message volume per 100 patients over time. The adjusted clinical message volume is depicted in Figure 2.6, and the nonclinical volume is shown in Figure 2.7.

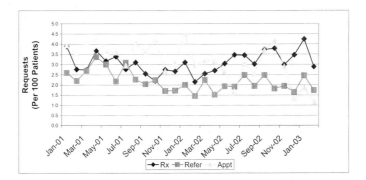

FIGURE 2.7. Administrative requests over time (prescription, referral, and appointment request).

We also examined patients' behavior in looking at their clinical record online. Every month, 16% of registered patients look at their record through PatientSite.

Discussion

Patients cannot register for PatientSite unless they have a physician who uses PatientSite. Once we enroll a physician, all of the physician's patients become eligible to use PatientSite. Since patients usually find out about PatientSite when they come to the office, the patients accrue gradually over time. Because of this, even if we stopped registering new physicians (which happened near the end of 2002 as we were doing a major system upgrade), we would continue to add new patients until we exhausted the panels of the registered physicians.

One of the things that worries physicians about electronic communication is that they will be flooded with e-mail. Our data do not support this concern. Looking at the volume of clinical messages, we see that the number of messages handled by physicians is quite modest, on the order of 20 to 40 messages per month per 100 patients. If we imagine a busy practitioner who has 1500 patients using PatientSite, the maximum number of messages he can expect to handle from patients each day would be 15.

Even as it has been well received by many patients and physicians, PatientSite has raised controversial issues that are worthy of future discussion:

- Should patients have full electronic access to their record? Should certain types of data be restricted? Is it necessary for physicians to review results before patients can view them?
- How should information from the medical record be presented to patients to enhance their understanding of their health without needlessly alarming them?
- PatientSite has three major stakeholder groups: patients, physicians, and practices. How can we best balance the needs and concerns of each group to guide development?
- Should patients be permitted to use PatientSite to view their record if their physician does not use PatientSite?
- For patients with more than one physician using PatientSite, how do we incorporate all the physicians' preferences about patient access to information?
- What should happen to patient-entered information in the personal health record? Should physicians be able to view the patient's personal health record? Should they be required to do so?
- In a teaching environment, how should preceptors oversee their trainees' use of electronic messaging with patients?
- Is it fair to offer a service like PatientSite to Internet-enabled patients without enhancing service for patients who cannot use the Internet?

- Should physicians be reimbursed for using PatientSite? If so, who should pay? How much should they be reimbursed?
- How can healthcare organizations justify the cost of projects like Patient-Site?

Conclusion

Online health consumers are increasingly prevalent and are therefore important to healthcare providers. Organizations must fulfill their needs for communication, information, convenience, and access to their health records. PatientSite is an excellent way to meet these needs. Both patients and providers have vigorously adopted it, yet the demand on physician time is modest. The system has introduced controversial and interesting issues that we continue to work through. PatientSite is also a useful platform for future projects, such as patient-computer interviewing, disease management, healthcare quality, and patient safety.

PatientSite can be accessed at https://patientsite.bidmc.harvard.edu.

References

1. Manhattan Research, LLC. CyberCitizen Health v2.0. New York: Manhattan Research, 2002.
2. Horrigan JB, Rainie L. Counting on the Internet. Washington, DC: ,Pew Internet and American Life Project, December 2002.
3. Harris Interactive. No significant change in the number of "cyber-chondriacs"—those who go online for health care information. Health Care News 2003;3:4.
4. Harris Interactive. Patient/physician online communication: many patients want it, would pay for it, and it would influence their choice of doctors and health plans. Health Care News 2002;2:8.
5. Manhattan Research, LLC. Taking the Pulse v2.0. New York: Manhattan Research, 2002.
6. Kane B, Sands DZ for the AMIA Internet Working Group, Task Force on Guidelines for the Use of Clinic-Patient Electronic Mail. Guidelines for the clinical use of electronic mail with patients. J Am Med Inform Assoc 1998;5:104–111.
7. Bleich HL, Beckley RF, Horowitz G, et al. Clinical computing in a teaching hospital. N Engl J Med 1985;312:756–764.
8. Safran C, Slack WV, Bleich HL. Role of computing in patient care in two hospitals. MD Comput 1989;6:41–48.
9. Safran C, Sands DZ, Rind DM. Online medical records: a decade of experience. Methods Inform Med 1999;38:308–312.
10. Slack WV, Slack CW. Patient-computer dialogue. N Engl J Med 1972;286:1304–1309.
11. Fishbach RL, Sionelo-Bayog A, Needle A, Delbanco TL. The patient and practitioner as co-authors of the medical record. Patient Couns Health Educ 1980;2(1):1–5.
12. Mukamal KJ, Smetana GW, Delbanco T. Clinicians, educators, and investigators in

general internal medicine: bridging the gaps. J Gen Intern Med 2002;17(7):565–571.

13. Clifford JC, Horvath J, eds. Advancing professional nursing practice: innovations and Boston's Beth Israel Hospital. New York: Springer, 1990.

14. Beatrice DF, Thomas CP, Biles B. Grant making with an impact: the Picker/Commonwealth Patient-Centered Care Program. Health Affairs 1998;17:236–244.

15. Kantz B, Wandel J, Fladger A, Folcarelli P, Burger S, Clifford JC. Developing patient and family education services: innovations for the changing healthcare environment. J Nurs Admin 1998;28:2,11–18.

16. Sands DZ, Halamka JD, Pellaton D. PatientSite: a Web-based clinical communication and health education tool. Health Information Management Systems Society annual conference, Chicago, 2001.

17. Halamka JD, Szolovits P, Rind D, Safran C. A WWW implementation of national recommendations for protecting electronic health information. J Am Med Inform Assoc 1997;4(6):458–464.

18. Masys DR, Baker DB. Patient-Centered Access to Secure Systems Online (PCASSO): 8a secure approach to clinical data access via the World Wide Web. Proc AMIA Annual Fall Symposium 1997;340–343.

19. http://www.rsasecurity.com/products/securid/tokens.html, 2003.

20. Slack WV, Bleich HL. The CCC system in two teaching hospitals: a progress report. Int J Med Inform 1999;54:183–196.

21. Slack WV. Cybermedicine: how computing empowers doctors and patients for better health care (revised and updated edition). San Francisco: Jossey-Bass, 2001.

3
HeartCare: A Scalable Technological Solution to the Challenges of Posthospitalization Recovery from CABG Surgery

PATRICIA FLATLEY BRENNAN, JOSETTE JONES,
SHIRLEY M.MOORE, AND CONNIE VISOVSKY

Patients recovering from coronary artery bypass graft (CABG) surgery face four key challenges in the posthospitalization stage: monitoring their progress toward healing, understanding the desirable and undesirable indicators of recovery, appraising their own body state, and acting in accord with the alignment of what was expected and what actually occurred. They must manage their own recovery protocol, integrating recommendations from clinicians regarding medications, wound care, and activity tolerance into a home routine. They must mend, or heal, following the prescribed activity/rest/nutrition guidelines to ensure both physiological healing as well as psychological recovery. Finally, they must be motivated to adopt new heart-healthy behaviors while avoiding those that interfere with healing and recovery.

To date, the discharge-teaching encounter served as the sole opportunity to prepare patients to actively engage in posthospital recovery routines. Yet the move toward short-stay hospitalizations coupled with the increasing diversity of information needs experienced by an increasingly older, more frail patient population challenges the ability of nurses to meet patients' information needs in an already-dense discharge planning routine.[1] Additionally, recent evidence of the value of personalized, tailored health information[2] necessitates a transition from providing patients with enumerations of best practices to facilitating patient access to personally relevant, staged health information resources. Innovative application of information technology could assist patients in the postdischarge phase of recovery from CABG surgery and facilitate their access to tailored recovery information.

Our team created HeartCare,[3] a browser-accessible health information system designed to assist home-dwelling patients in the recovery from CABG surgery. HeartCare was built on the established evidence that patient self-management of complex health situations benefits from communication with peers[4] and professionals[5] and timely access to relevant, personally tailored health information.[6] This chapter describes the HeartCare system, examining the knowledge resource, communication utilities, technical platform, nursing role, and patient experience. We conclude with comments regarding scalability of these innovations.

The HeartCare System

HeartCare consists of a set of Internet-accessible, browser-viewed information resources; tailoring algorithms; and communication, tailoring, storage, and data management utilities. A key component of HeartCare is the daily presence of an advanced practice nurse (author C.V.), who oversaw content development, posted or responded to messages from participants, and observed key behavioral indicators of recovery, such as posting or other types of participation. HeartCare was created as an experimental system that served as part of a field evaluation of home-based telehealth interventions, funded by the National Library of Medicine (LM) and the National Institute of Nursing Research (LM grant 6249; P.F. Brennan, principal investigator).

The HeartCare Server

The HeartCare server included a message library, the algorithms for matching messages to individuals, and communication resources. Microsoft Web Server served as our implementation platform; an NT device linked within a secure network, and mirrored off-site, served as the technical platform.

The message library included an index to more than 400 HTML-marked-up files that addressed the full range of cardiac recovery information needed by patients.[7] Consistent with our design philosophy of reuse and sustainability, we selected, evaluated, indexed, and held the addresses for information resources that already existed on the Internet. Where such information resources were lacking, we created files to meet selected patient needs, such as resuming sexual activity, pain management specific to women recovering from CABG surgery, and family dynamics. Our selection and creation of information resources was guided by Johnson's framework, which advises that patients do best with health information that explains what to expect and how to manage the recovery experience.[8]

The content of the knowledge resources was organized around the four phases of recovery from CABG surgery, roughly lasting from discharge through the 6-month anniversary. In the first 2 weeks, content focused on the symptom management aspects of recovery. During the next 3 weeks, the content focus shifted to resumption of physical activity. In the subsequent 6 weeks, knowledge resources targeted return to prior function. Finally, for the last 3 months of the recovery period, content addressed health behavior modification.

An efficient matching algorithm, and one that could have been implemented automatically through the HeartCare server, was key to providing tailored health information to participants (Fig. 3.1). Our staff (J.J.) created and implemented, in Access, a matching algorithm that required three components: First, each of

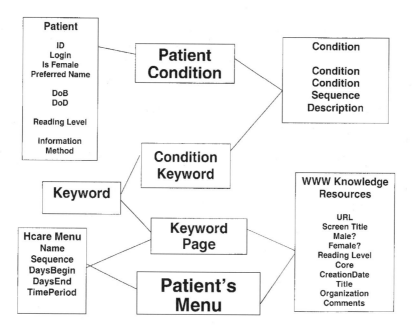

FIGURE 3.1. The matching algorithm.

the 400+ Web resources needed to be tagged with its relevance to the point of recovery and its pertinence to key aspects of CABG recovery, such as gender of the patient, comorbidities, and lifestyle issues. Second, a descriptor for each participant that included appraisal of the patient on these tailoring variables had to be created. Third, a mechanism for matching the participant at a specific point in time to the information resources was needed to ensure that only information resources relevant to the particular participant at a given point in time were presented to the participant.

Three communication resources were made available to participants: a public bulletin board where participants could post messages to others in the HeartCare experiment and read messages from others; private electronic mail that permitted participants to interact with each other; and a private "mail to the nurse" function that allowed the participant to directly communicate with the nurses. All messaging services permitted free-text entries and lacked any special characters or HTML coding. Project staff did not read or review participants' e-mail to each other; a project nurse accessed the "mail to the nurse" utility and the public messaging system daily to monitor discussions and to contribute clarification or information as requested.

Some management utilities were created to support the HeartCare system; others served the research data collection operations of the project. Participant access to the time-sequenced tailored information for one's care occurred through a series of active server pages that were evoked each time a participant accessed the HeartCare system. These pages permitted secure identification of the participant, initiated an encounter-logging feature, and ensured the presentation of health information relevant to the participant at the specific point of recovery.

We employed WebTrends™ to facilitate monitoring server operations, facilitate link checking, and create use data reports. A pager-activation function of WebTrends could notify technical staff when the server malfunctioned. Because of the reliance on external Web resources as part of our message library, a link-checking mechanism was employed to ensure the integrity of the links to information resources and to allow for removal or modification of links no longer valid. Finally, review of information processing (IP) access to our HeartCare server permitted detection of any inappropriate access and provided confirmation of the security of the system.

Nursing Practice in the HeartCare Environment

The presence of an advanced practice nurse was an integral part of the HeartCare project. An advanced practice nurse (C.V.), aided by additional nursing and health communications staff, guided the selection of information resources for the message library. In addition, the research team worked with the nurse to create practice protocols, including how to respond to requests for emergency interventions, appropriate referral policies, and what to do about participants who did not access the system for long periods of time.

The advanced practice nurse served as the primary communicator with participants, receiving messages through the "mail to the nurse" utility. Her interactions with patients were guided by professional judgment as well as her clinical experience in symptom interpretation and patient teaching. Interaction with the nurse occurred almost exclusively in the electronic environment.

HeartCare: The Participants' Experience

Accessing HeartCare

Participants accessed the HeartCare server via WebTV™ devices provided to them by a research project underwriting the development and evaluation of the HeartCare system. WebTV is a set-top device that employs a proprietary browser to display HTML-coded files on a standard television set. Connection to the Internet is made via standard telephone lines. All participants had at least 6 months' access to HeartCare. Project staff set up all participant-specific resources, delivered equipment to the participant's home, and provided a 90-minute training session.

Participants could access the HeartCare service 24 hours a day. Participants first logged in with a private user identification, selected by the participant. Access to some functions, such as private mail, required a second-level identification check. Once the participant had accessed the HeartCare system, utilities on the server selected and displayed menus linked to specific information resources through a process that required noting the participant's identity, recording the participant's profile, determining how much time had passed since discharge, and evoking the matching algorithm. This process occurred sufficiently fast that participants were unaware of any delays. Once authorization and profiling were complete, a set of menu-accessible pages was presented to the participant.

Participants accessed the HeartCare system about 48 times over the course of their 6-month participation, accessing the system two to three times a week in the early discharge period and about once a week in the later period (3 to 6 months after discharge). About half of the participants accessed the system regularly throughout the 6-month period. Participant access to the information resources on HeartCare varied widely, with some participants accessing quite a large number of the pages in the message library and others accessing almost none. No obvious relationship between frequency of encounter and frequency of access to information was evident. On most occasions participants used one or both of the communication services (public bulletin board or private e-mail). About half of the patients accessed private e-mail more often than the public bulletin board.

Evaluating HeartCare

We evaluated HeartCare in a randomized field experiment that involved about 150 patients recovering from CABG surgery. Patients who were deemed eligible to participate in an experimental 6-month evaluation of HeartCare were recruited in-hospital on the third or fourth day after surgery. Of these patients, 55 were randomized to the HeartCare intervention, and 47 actually received the intervention in their homes. (The remainder experienced problems postsurgery that subsequently made them ineligible for participation in the study.) We compared participants with access to HeartCare to those who used a standard audiotaped coaching program. Preliminary findings indicate that participants find HeartCare helpful and feasible to use in the early discharge period.

What Is Needed to Make Interventions Like HeartCare Scalable?

The growth in health applications on the Internet suggests that patients find these interventions helpful and valuable at many points in the recovery process. However, as noted the Pew Foundation's study of the Internet and American Life,[9] while people are generally happy with their ability to access health information on the Internet, they express frustration and dismay with specific instances of seeking particular health information. Strategies are needed that better understand the health information needs of individuals, and that employ this understanding to more efficiently and accurately link participants to the specific information they require.

Most Internet-based health information resources fall into one of two categories: those built by a particular institution, like a hospital or clinic, wherein the content closely reflects the practice structure and clinical processes delivered by that clinic; and those developed for the general public, wherein the content is likely to encompass all aspects that experts in the domain view as relevant. Few systems have the capability to present information tailored any more specifically than on the specific topic that the individual has identified. Furthermore, the information presented may be redundant or even in conflict with information accessible in the person's local environment. Therefore, scalability of Internet-based interventions require greater understanding of the successful strategies already employed by patients as they manage health information, and alignment of the health information presented on the Internet with that available in the individual's community.

Finally, reliance on Internet-based health information presumes the existence of a technical infrastructure sufficient to support the secure delivery of health information in many formats. Ensuring that a robust health information infrastructure exists in all communities in the United States represents a challenge that cannot be ignored by those who hope that the Internet-based health services will complement and extend those already available in our healthcare delivery system.

Conclusion

The HeartCare system stands as a successful demonstration of a technological solution to the challenge of postdischarge recovery from CABG surgery. Participants found the system acceptable and relevant to their recovery experience. Scalability of solutions like HeartCare require careful attention to understanding patients' health information needs, evaluation of the individual and community resources for health information management, and assurance that the technical infrastructure for success exists in all communities.

References

1. Penque S, Petersen B, Arom K, Ratner E, Halm M. Early discharge with home health care in the coronary artery bypass patient. Dimens Crit Care Nurs 1999;18(6):40–48.
2. Ryan P, Lauver D. Tailored health messages: do they really work? J Nursing Scholarship 2003.
3. Brennan PF, Moore SM, Bjornsdottir G, Jones J, Visovsky C, Rogers M. HeartCare: an Internet-based information and support system for patient home recovery after coronary artery bypass graft (CABG) surgery. J Adv Nurs 2001;35(5):699–708.

4. Parent N, Fortin F. A randomized, controlled trial of vicarious experience through peer support for male first-time cardiac surgery patients: impact on anxiety, self-efficacy expectation, and self-reported activity. Heart Lung: J Acute Crit Care 2000;29(6):389–400.
5. Savage LS, Grap MJ. Telephone monitoring after early discharge for cardiac surgery patients. Am J Crit Care 1999;8(3):154–159.
6. Kreuter MW, Strecher VJ, Glassman B. One size does not fit all: the case for tailoring print materials. Ann Behav Med 1999;21(4):276–283.
7. Moore SM, Visovsky C, Brennan PF, et al. (In progress.)
8. Johnson JE. Self-regulation theory and coping with physical illness. Res NursHealth 1999;22(6):435–448.
9. Pew Foundation. The Internet and American life. Philadelphia: Pew Foundation, 2002.

4
A Clinic in Every Home

BONNIE J. WAKEFIELD AND MICHAEL G. KIENZLE

Imagine an entire population with access at home to a network that enables people to access information, communicate with providers and other interested parties, and receive some diagnostic and therapeutic services. The home, as a site of healthcare delivery, is of increasing interest to healthcare planners and providers. For those individuals whose access to traditional healthcare delivery is limited by circumstances such as distance and mobility, home-delivered services would be particularly attractive and potentially beneficial. In recent years, major advances in computing and telecommunications technologies, particularly the exponential growth of the Internet, have suggested possible approaches to improving health through the direct provision of services to patients.

Telehealth research and development has been an area of intense interest at the University of Iowa and the Iowa City Veterans Administration Medical Center for nearly a decade. Our research has been supported by a variety of state and federal agencies, including the Agency for Healthcare Research and Quality (AHRQ), General Services Administration, Veterans Administration, and most notably the National Library of Medicine. We have studied the utility of a variety of telehealth applications aimed at vulnerable populations such as rural trauma victims, disabled children, and underserved patients with mental illness. In recent years, we have become more focused on healthcare services (education, monitoring, and support) delivered directly to patients in the home or other residential settings.

This chapter briefly describes the evidence supporting home telehealth, offers a simple conceptual model for Internet-delivered health services, and describes some of our own research and experience that we believe support the achievability of the model we have described.

The Current Evidence Base for Home Telehealth

Telehealth holds great promise in increasing access to high-quality health care, enhancing patient satisfaction, and managing resource utilization. Although more than 300 telehealth programs have been implemented nationwide, there is little empirical evidence supporting the efficacy and cost-effectiveness of telehealth, as most of the literature on telehealth is descriptive and anecdotal in nature. This section reviews the current evidence base for telehealth home care.

Four reviews have been published describing telehealth research across a wide range of patient populations. These reviews have addressed telephone-based health care,[1] patient satisfaction with interactive video consultation,[2] and clinical trials in home- and office-based care.[3,4]

The first review[1] summarized, categorized, and evaluated randomized controlled trials evaluating distance-medicine technologies. Of the 80 trials reviewed, seven used computerized communications and 73 used telephone-based communication. Of these 80 trials, 61 (76%) were studies in which the provider initiated the communication with patients and 50 (63%) reported positive outcomes or benefits. Based on this review, the investigators concluded there were significant benefits for distance medical care in the areas of immunizations and vaccination rates, mammography rates, glucose levels and diet in people with diabetes, lifestyle changes during cardiac rehabilitation programs, and pain and function in patients with osteoarthritis. Reviewed studies showed mixed results in the effect of distance medicine in tobacco-use prevention. For the most part, studies did not address costs or cost effectiveness of the intervention.

A second review focused on patient satisfaction with telehealth.[2] Studies were identified through a computerized search of the literature covering 1966 to 1998. Clinical trials that explored patient satisfaction with real-time interactive video consultation were included in the review. Of the 32 studies included in the review, three were studies of home-based telehealth. These three studies had relatively small sample sizes ($n = 3, 20, 22$). Most studies were demonstrations or feasibility studies, and thus exhibited a number of methodological deficiencies, including small convenience samples, lack of a control group, and use of investigator-developed instruments to measure satisfaction. While patients were generally satisfied with this mode of interaction in the studies reviewed, important issues were not addressed, including lack of attention to the reasons patients are satisfied or dissatisfied and failure to address how the interactive video consultation affected patient–provider communication.

The third review was conducted by Hersh and colleagues[4] under a contract from the AHRQ. A similar review was conducted by Currell and colleagues.[3] Since all studies reviewed by Currell et al were included in the Hersh review, only the report by Hersh is discussed here. This review evaluated the efficacy of telehealth interventions for health outcomes in two classes of applications: home-based and office/hospital-based. The investigators searched major electronic databases covering the years 1966 to 2000; reviewed telehealth reports, compilations, and three systematic reviews different in scope from their study; identified articles from reference lists; contacted known telehealth experts; and hand-searched the two major telehealth journals. Over 4000 references were identified. Applying the inclusion criteria yielded 19 articles on home-based telehealth. The strongest evidence for efficacy of telehealth relative to clinical outcomes comes from management of chronic disease, hypertension, and AIDS. While the most studied area is diabetes, these investigators found the benefits inconclusive when hemoglobin $HgbA_{1c}$ levels were used as the outcome measure.

In conclusion, the current evidence on home-based telehealth shows mixed results in terms of outcomes. In general, the cost-effectiveness of home-based telehealth is not addressed in studies. Patient satisfaction is high, but studies are descriptive and the reasons patients like (or do not like) home telehealth have not been explored. Providers are more resistant to using the technology, but reasons for this have not been elucidated. There are few telehealth-specific outcome measures available to evaluate the efficacy of these technologies. The future research agenda must address the following: which populations will benefit most from home telehealth; appropriate matching of patient need to technology; adequate sample sizes to make definitive statements regarding the efficacy of the home-based application; patient safety issues; the mechanism of effect, i.e., why home telehealth works; and organizational infrastructure needed to support telehealth services.

The Clinic in Every Home Model

For home-based telehealth to become a reality, the questions identified in the previous section must be answered. We explored some of these questions through the Clinic in Every Home (CIEH) project, which developed a model consisting of three distinct layers, shown schematically in Figure 4.1.

The base layer, content, represents access to personalized information specific to each user depending on age, gender, medical history or interests, and (importantly) place of residence. This would permit dissemination of important public health information (air and water quality, cancer statistics, etc.) and reporting of potentially important information from each home (epidemics, bioterrorism events, etc.). Two applications that illustrate the content layer of the model, the Virtual Hospital® and the network interface developed for the CIEH project, are described in a subsequent section of this chapter.

The middle layer, communication, consists of a secure messaging system that would permit structured communication with providers and support groups.

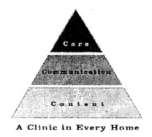

A Clinic in Every Home

FIGURE 4.1. A Clinic in Every Home model.

Four projects that explore issues surrounding the communication layer of the model are described in a subsequent section of this chapter: a diabetes education and support project, two studies comparing platforms for telehealth home care, and a survey of physicians about use of e-mail consultations.

The top level, care, implies a more interactive functionality that permits limited diagnosis and management of chronic or some acute healthcare problems. This layer is the most problematic in terms of widespread availability due to cost, technical complexity, lack of adequate bandwidth available to the general public, and the clinical management challenges that such a system would create. Several projects that illustrate the feasibility of providing care in a patient's home are subsequently described, including Resource Link of Iowa, the provision of specialist clinics to residents in a long-term-care setting, and community-based telehealth programs using a variety of home-based technologies.

Content Layer: The University of Iowa's Virtual Hospital

The content layer of our CIEH model is imagined as a personalized, relevant, accurate, and usable source of information over the Internet. While there are many sources of health information for providers and consumers on the Internet, much has been written about the shortcomings found at many of these sites.[5]-[7] Most of the healthcare sites currently meeting these requirements noted above are sponsored by government agencies (MedlinePlus from the National Library of Medicine is a good example), nonprofit health-focused organizations (American Heart Association, American Diabetes Association), and universities (OncoLink from the University of Pennsylvania). At the University of Iowa (UI), our approach and philosophy have been significantly shaped by our experience as the publisher of the Virtual Hospital, a multimedia library designed for use by healthcare providers and their patients.

The Virtual Hospital (VH) began in 1991 as a small collection of digital textbooks prepared by interested UI faculty. The collection appeared on the Internet in 1992 as a Gopher site, and moved to the World Wide Web (WWW) late in 1993 as the (approximately) 250th WWW site in existence (http://www.vh.org). From 1994 to 1997 the collection rapidly expanded due to support from the National Library of Medicine. Since 1997, the ongoing site production has been supported as a public service of the UI Carver College of Medicine and the UI Hospitals and Clinics. In the decade since the VH first appeared on the Web, it has grown dramatically in several dimensions: collection size (Virtual Children's Hospital and Virtual Naval Hospital have been added), utilization (in 2002, there were 106 million qualified "hits" and 42 million pages read by over 10 million visitors), global reach (25% of use is from outside the United States, in part through four mirror sites worldwide), and recognition (Scientific American Sci/Tech Web Award 2001 is one recent example). The success of the VH is attributable to a multitude of factors, a number of which have been reviewed by the group responsible for the creation of the site.[8] By successfully negotiating a number of challenges related to digital content ownership, site management, mirroring, translation, archiving, and user interactions, the resulting Web site is a publicly supported resource that meets many of the requirements for a ubiquitous health network. A key element required under the CIEH model still remains to be accomplished, however. True personalization of the VH site will require the dynamic generation of pages using a different database design from that currently in use.

Network Interface Development

As part of the CIEH project, we created a prototype demonstration site to facilitate focus group and other discussions of how a personalized Internet health portal might work. The prototype featured a simple three-step process for public participation, consisting of a registration process that created a user name and password and captured enough information to allow integration of local, age, and gender-specific information while permitting anonymity (Fig. 4.2). The consumer then personalized the portal by selecting medical problems of interest and other information resources unrelated directly to health (weather, hobbies, etc.) (Fig. 4.3). Completion of this simple process dynamically generated a single screen on which the user could access a host of personalized resources, including access to secure messaging with healthcare providers

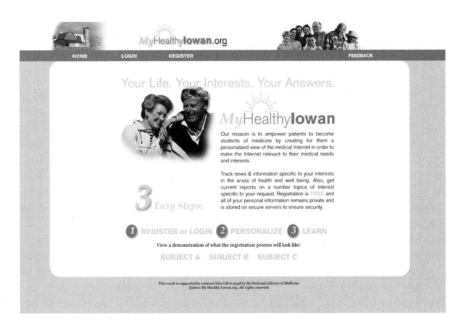

FIGURE 4.2. Registration page. Available at http://www.myhealthyiowan.org. (Reprinted with permission.)

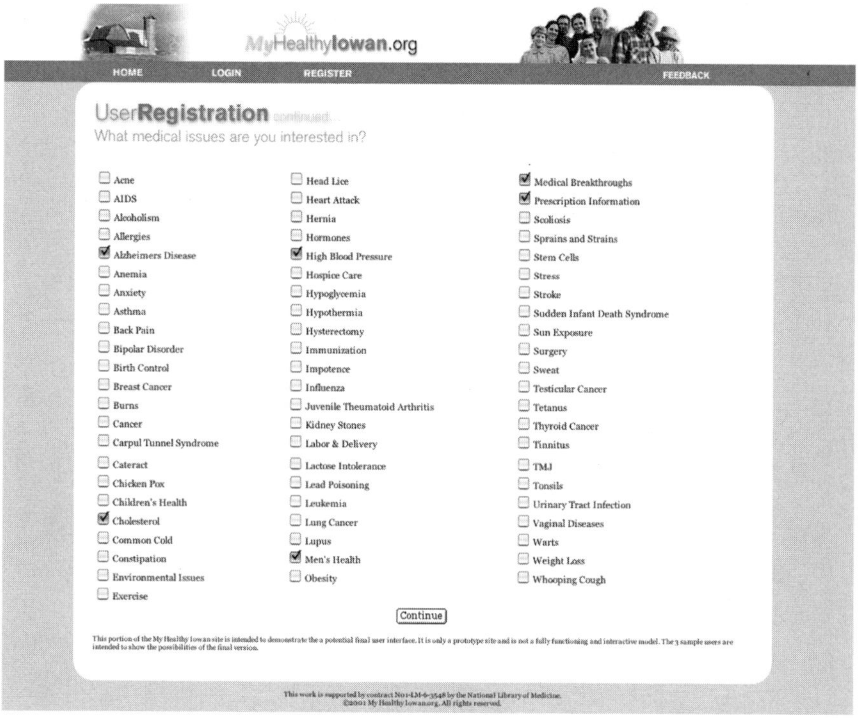

FIGURE 4.3. User personalization selections. Available at http://www.myhealthyiowan.org. (Reprinted with permission.)

and support groups (Fig. 4.4). The prototype is currently viewable at http://www.myhealthyiowan.org.

Communication Layer

This section provides a brief overview of a set of studies aimed at understanding factors that affect acceptance and use of educational and healthcare resources delivered by computer-based technology. Four studies are reported. The first three assess patient-technology interaction. The first evaluates the effect of Internet access to education and support on diabetes clinical outcomes. The next two studies compare user perceptions of ease of use and effectiveness between an Internet appliance and a computer, and compare a plain old telephone service (POTS)-based and Internet-based platform on nurse and patient preference, acceptance, and ease of use of two home video appliances. The fourth study describes a physician survey addressing the attitudes of physicians related to use of secure e-mail for patient consultation.

Internet Access to Education and Support in Diabetes

There is a very strong rationale for enhancing diabetes education, based on studies demonstrating a reduction in complications of diabetes through opti-

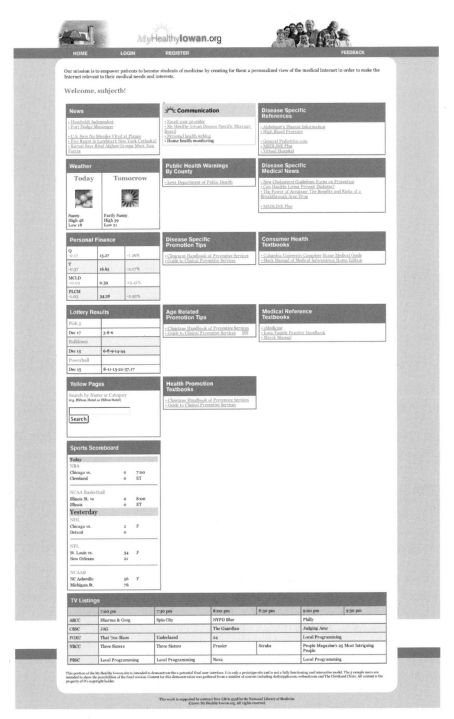

FIGURE 4.4. Personalized Web page. Available at http://www.myhealthyiowan.org. (Reprinted with permission.)

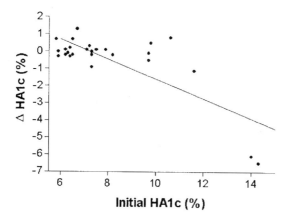

FIGURE 4.5. Percent change in hemoglobin HgbA$_{1c}$ levels associated with computer use.

mal glycemic control.[9] Patient education is an important component of management of diabetes,[10] but in many communities diabetes educators are not readily available. Expanding access to diabetes education over the Internet offers a potential means to provide ongoing diabetes education to large numbers of people. We examined the effect of providing Internet access, specialized resources, training, and support to adults with diabetes upon diabetes knowledge and a physiologic marker of glycemic control, HgbA$_{1c}$.

Thirty adults (15 men and 15 women), ranging in age from 19 to 83 years (mean 51), managed in a rural setting, with known type 1 or type 2 diabetes, matched for gender and body mass index, were randomly assigned to either receive (group I) or not receive (group II) an Apple iMac computer with Internet access for 3 months. A specially designed Web site was available where subjects could take advantage of diabetes education links; e-mail connections to other patients, participating providers, and technical support; and a threaded discussion forum. Training was provided to patients before starting Internet-based education. After 3 months, subjects crossed over to the opposite assignment. Diabetes knowledge tests consisting of 40 multiple-choice questions were administered; HgbA$_{1c}$ was measured; and weight and body mass index was determined before, at crossover, and at the end of the study. Diabetes knowledge showed a modest but statistically significant increase as a result of random assignment to Internet availability, including a Web site focused on diabetes education, but for the entire group there was no statistically significant improvement in glycemic control associated with the incremental knowledge. Interestingly, there was a significant positive correlation (p <.001, $r^2 = 0.59$) between improvement in HgbA$_{1c}$ before and after Internet availability and initial (prerandomization) HgbA$_{1c}$ levels (Fig. 4.5).

This study may suggest that more intense methods for computer-assisted instruction, beyond availability per se, may be required (e.g., an information prescription). Alternately, the study may have lacked power to detect a significant improvement in HgbA$_{1c}$, particularly among those subjects in reasonable control at study initiation. We were encouraged that a project of this type could be carried out in a rural community setting.

Comparison of Ease of Use Between an Internet Appliance and Computer

Computer-based patient education is a promising area of interest in health informatics. Increasing use of and access to the Internet and its resources suggests significant opportunities for patient education and disease management. However, realizing this potential is highly dependent on the interaction between the information seeker and the computer resource. While use of the Internet is growing rapidly, many individuals have very limited or no access to the network and little experience with computers. Internet appliances (devices designed for simplicity of use and functionality limited to Internet access) are available for those unfamiliar or uncomfortable with traditional computers. Whether these appliances are adequate for educational uses has not been explored.

Fifty medically unscreened subjects (16 males and 34 females; 36% between 61 and 70 years of age) were recruited from the volunteer program of the UI hospitals and clinics. Subjects evaluated the Apple iMac and Sony WebTV for a number of user characteristics including searching, navigating, scrolling, e-mail, print size and clarity, image clarity, and screen color and brightness. All subjects evaluated both devices, and subjects were randomized to start either with the iMac or the WebTV. After evaluating the features of both, subjects indicated a preference for one or the other, or no preference.

As a group, the volunteer subjects were fairly frequent users of computers and Internet access, with 70% using a computer more than 10 times per month and 54% using the Internet more than 10 times per month; 56% described themselves as being "very comfortable" using a computer. Users strongly preferred the iMac for searching, clarity, and screen color and brightness. Reported use of the computer more than 10 times per month was significantly related to preferences.

User perceptions of ease of use and effectiveness will play a role in the growth of the Internet for the education and management of patients with complex health problems. Not all devices used to access the Internet are perceived as equivalent, and the differences may have important implications for their use in healthcare settings. Internet appliances appear to be adequate for basic text and electronic mail functions, but may lack sufficient resolution and graphical quality for other educational functions, especially for more experienced computer users. Many patients have relatively little experience with computers and Internet access, but given training, tools, and access find these resources valuable and incorporate them into information-seeking about their disease.

Nurse and Patient Perceptions of Two Video Platforms for Delivery of Home Care

As noted earlier, evaluations of the effectiveness of care delivered to the home via interactive video has received limited attention. A wide variety of home telehealth monitoring devices has been developed, yet studies have not evaluated the effect of video on patient-provider communication or preferences of the end users (i.e., nurses and patients) for different models or types of home care technology. The purpose of this study was to compare the quality of nurse-patient interaction using two different video platforms designed for tele-home care. One platform used existing telephone lines (POTS) and the other used the Internet protocol (IP). Twenty-six nurses and 18 volunteer-simulated patients participated. Nurse-patient dyads completed scripted interactions on each video platform, followed by questionnaires assessing communication, acceptance, and preferences; 84% of participants ($n = 37$) preferred IP and 13% ($n = 6$) preferred POTS. Nurses and patients did not differ in overall preference. IP was rated significantly higher in all communication quality and acceptance areas except self-consciousness/embarrassment, ease of use, time required, and perceived expense of visit. Overall, 59% of participants would prefer in-person visits, and 23% would prefer video visits. Choosing between more frequent video visits and less frequent in-home visits, 75% preferred more frequent video visits, 18% preferred less frequent in-home visits. Patient ratings of both platforms were generally higher than nurses' ratings. Patients were more willing to use and recommend interactive video as a replacement for in-home nursing visits.

Physician Use of E-mail Consultation

The participation of members of the healthcare team in the provision of services online is a key variable in the success of our CIEH model. National studies as well as our own have repeatedly demonstrated considerable unfulfilled demand for e-mail access to physicians and other providers. To date, physicians have been slow to embrace electronic communication with their patients, although the vast majority both have and use Internet access, and report using e-mail to communicate with colleagues on clinical issues.

In recent months, reports have suggested an increased interest in providing online communication and consultation using secure messaging systems that also permit a number of other functions, which include billing for certain types of interactions, prescription management, communication with other office staff for appointments, and liability risk management through carefully crafted conditions of service. Several pilot studies supported by insurers[11-13] have suggested that a number of low-level, low-risk services can be provided online with acceptable outcomes, with high acceptance by providers and their patients.

To assess UI medical staff members' perceptions about and interest in using e-mail to communicate with their patients, we solicited their participation in a brief online survey in June 2002. Of 298 surveys sent, 132 usable surveys (44%) were returned. Respondents' age distribution was as follows: 12% were 40 years of age or younger; 46% were 41 to 50; 30% were 51 to 60; and 12% were 61 or older. Two questions focused on physicians' current use of e-mail. Regarding frequency of use, 14% ($n = 19$) frequently use e-mail; 28% ($n = 37$) sometimes use e-mail; 45% ($n = 59$) rarely use e-mail; and 13% ($n = 17$) have never used e-mail to communicate with patients. The current overall perspec-

TABLE 4.1. Factors positively influencing physicians' use of e-mail with patients (n = 132 respondents).

Item	Number responding yes
Reduces need for follow-up phone calls	93 (70%)
More effective and timely communication with patients enhances care	90 (68%)
Documentation of the exchange of information	64 (48%)
Ability to easily share electronic messages with colleagues and office staff	53 (40%)
Electronic e-mail access is valued by my patients	51 (39%)
Ability to attach additional information to e-mail or easily direct patients to other online resources	23 (17%)

tive about use of e-mail with patients was that 42% (n = 55) have a positive perspective on physician-patient e-mail communication; 33% (n = 44) have a neutral perspective; and 25% (n = 33) have a negative perspective. Factors that positively or negatively influenced use of e-mail communication with patients are listed in Tables 4.1 and 4.2. Sixty-eight percent of respondents indicated an interest in participating in a pilot project involving a standardized secure messaging and consultation system.

We believe that considerable interest exists on the part of both patients and their providers, and that electronic messaging will become an important tool in the near term, particularly as systems that address the concerns voiced

TABLE 4.2. Factors negatively influencing physicians' use of e-mail with patients (n = 132 respondents).

Item	Number responding yes
Current or potential volume of e-mail messages time required	101 (77%)
Risk of liability	66 (50%)
Lack of security of current e-mail systems	65 (49%)
Lack of easy integration with patients' medical records paper or electronic	57 (43%)
Lack of reimbursement for use of e-mail with patients	52 (39%)
Belief that patients prefer phone or face-to-face interactions	21 (16%)
Nature of my practice makes e-mail communication inappropriate	17 (13%)
Lack of familiarity or experience with computers and basic applications	1 (<1%)

by physicians are developed and refined, and providers learn how to work online communication with patients into their daily work flow.

Care Layer

This layer reports on a set of applications that illustrate the care component of the CIEH model. The first subsection describes Resource Link of Iowa, the second describes delivery of specialty services to residents of a long-term-care setting, and the third describes a large-scale implementation of a technology-facilitated home care program using a variety of technologies across a broad range of patient populations.

Resource Link of Iowa

Since January 1998, an in-home video approach has been used to manage the care of chronically ill patients throughout the state of Iowa. Resource Link of Iowa (RLI) uses a POTS-based video system (referred to as a videophone) that supports a two-way interactive audio/video connection between a base station and a remote (home) unit using a standard telephone line. The base station is composed of a Pentium computer, two monitors (computer and television), and a camera kit—a piece of equipment that combines a telephone, microphone, and video camera.

The three-piece home unit consists of a 13-inch color monitor, a camera kit, and a remote control device similar to a television remote. To establish online contact, the base station operator activates the system, and the user of the home unit responds by pushing the Start button on the remote control device. During the online visit, the base station operator and the participant at home see and talk to each other, with all functions controlled at the base station. When the visit is completed the participant presses the End Call button on the remote.

Patients have been selected for home telehealth visits using one or more of the following criteria:

- High utilization of hospital or office visits
- Chronic or select acute illness
- Adequate cognitive ability of patient or caregiver
- Understanding of program and desire for improved health status
- Endorsement of personal physician
- Good match between patient need and delivery model (teaching, supervising, prevention, practice)
- Patient has a home phone
- Patient is able to move or be moved

Through the end of 2002, 139 patients had been cared for using this system. Patients lived in 76 of Iowa's 99 counties (Fig. 4.6). Many patients lived as far away as 250 miles from the base station. Installation of equipment and initial

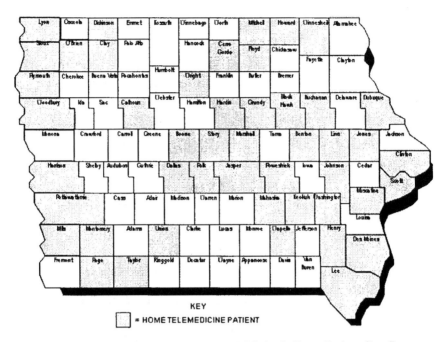

KEY

☐ = HOME TELEMEDICINE PATIENT

FIGURE 4.6. University of Iowa Hospitals and Clinics Indigent Patient Care Program: home telemedicine patient distribution, 1998 to November 2002. (Source: Report to the Iowa Legislature, 2003. Reprinted with permission.)

training was accomplished through a cooperative agreement between RLI and the community-based units of the Visiting Nurses Association. Of these 139 patients, 111 were enrolled through the Iowa Indigent Care Program, a support program that provides virtually all outpatient and inpatient care provided at the UI hospitals and clinics, including transportation, lodging, and prescriptions. As such, it presented a unique opportunity to estimate the impact of home telehealth visits after introducing the intervention in this population. We were able to determine utilization and cost of care for equal numbers of months before and after the initiation of home telehealth visits in 1999, 2000, and 2001. The findings were

TABLE 4.3. Pre- and post-home telehealth comparison for aggregate admissions and outpatient visits.

	Pre-home telehealth	Post-home telehealth	Percent change
Admissions	606	495	-18.3%
Outpatient visits	2457	2161	-12.0%

NOTE: Comparison based on equal time periods pre and post starting on home telehealth (n = 111).

reasonably consistent from year to year. Generally, two thirds of patients had fewer combined outpatient and inpatient visits, while roughly one third had more combined visits, when compared to an equivalent lead-in period prior to initiation of home telehealth visits. Our aggregate experience is shown in Table 4.3 and demonstrates a 21.6% reduction in admissions to the UI hospitals and a 12% reduction in UI outpatient visits.

A substantial cost avoidance was realized for the Indigent Care Program appropriation while providing a highly satisfactory service to enrollees, many of whom lived in remote parts of the state and had no prior experience with technology of this type. The ease of operation, immediate access to the service through POTS, and collaborative arrangements with community home nursing providers have been notable success factors.

Long-Term Care

Approximately 43% of all U.S. residents will spend some time in a nursing home during their lives.[14] Nursing home residents have high rates of chronic illness and disability. For example, 80% are mobility dependent and require a device or individual to assist them with ambulation. Paradoxically, relatively few physicians routinely make patient care visits in nursing homes. Thus, the frail elderly in nursing homes must frequently travel to receive specialty services. A major potential benefit of telehealth in long-term care (LTC) is greater and timelier access to specialized services that are not available within the facility where the patient resides. This series of studies evaluated the provision of specialty services via interactive video to residents in a large, multi-level, LTC setting. Two studies are described in this section: a nurse-managed chronic wound clinic and provision of specialty physician services to residents in an LTC setting.

Chronic wounds, such as pressure ulcers, diabetic foot ulcers, venous ulcers, and arterial ulcers, are a common problem among older persons. Proper management of chronic wounds requires frequent, routine monitoring of the wound-healing progress to optimize healing and ensure early recognition of impending complications. This project evaluated the implementation of a nurse-managed telehealth chronic wound clinic for residents of one LTC facility. Prior to implementation of the clinic, the wound consultant was making a 150-mile round trip to the LTC facility to consult with facility staff on the management of chronic wounds. Because of the distance, the consultant's trips to the facility were irregular. The objectives for implementing the telehealth chronic wound clinic included reducing travel costs and time for the consultant and timelier follow-up for patients. Data were collected from patients at the LTC facility, seven primary nurses and one skin care nurse at the LTC facility, and two consultant nurses providing telehealth wound assessment. Analyses compared on-site and telehealth assessments for 13 individual wound consultations. Interrater reliability for nine different wound characteristics ranged from 54% to 100%.[15] The cost of telehealth wound consultations was estimated to be $92.80 for each 20-minute consultation.[16] Data were also collected from the nurses and LTC residents on satisfaction with the telehealth clinic compared to in-person assessments.[17] The LTC residents found the telehealth consultation to be as good as the in-person assessment, although patients noted difficulty hearing and seeing the telehealth consultant. Nurses were equally satisfied with both the telehealth and in-person consultations and felt both consultation modes were a productive use of their time and skills.

A second study evaluated the provision of specialty physician clinic visits via interactive video to residents at the same facility. Specifically, we assessed physician, nurse, and patient satisfaction with the visit and outcomes of the consultation. Data were collected on 75 individual patient consultations. Most of these were follow-up visits (97%, $n = 73$) in urology, neurology, cardiology, and general surgery clinics. The most frequent clinical outcome was a change in treatment plan without a need to schedule a face-to-face visit ($n = 32$, 43%), or no change in treatment ($n = 21$, 28%). Physicians ratings of the telehealth consultations were for the most part positive: 76% good to excellent for usefulness in developing a diagnosis; 85% good to excellent for usefulness in developing a treatment plan; 76% good to excellent for quality of transmission; and 84% good to excellent for satisfaction with the consult format. Overall patient acceptance of telehealth services was high: 72% of patients were satisfied with the consult format, while 8% were neutral and only 6% were somewhat dissatisfied (14% did not respond to this question). All the patients (100%) believed the specialist understood their problem, while 92% felt it was easier to get medical care via telehealth.

Veterans Administration Community Care Coordination Service

Our belief in the CIEH model is strengthened by additional work ongoing in the Veterans Administration (VA). One of the largest evaluations to date of technology-facilitated home care is being conducted by the Department of Veterans Affairs in Florida.[18] Since April 2000, almost 800 veterans have been enrolled in the Florida VA Network 8 Community Care Coordination Service (CCCS). The CCCS integrates the care coordinator role with technology. Technologies are chosen based on patient needs and include videophones with and without peripheral devices, in-home messaging devices (i.e., Health Buddy), and instamatic cameras for weekly photographs of wounds. During the planning process, program managers found that 4% of patients in the network consumed over 40% of patient care resources. Thus, the service focuses on those patients who are frail, medically complex patients and high users of services. Using this model, patients who received the care management and technology intervention had substantially fewer clinic visits (26% lower), emergent visits (29% lower), hospital admissions (55% lower), and nursing home days of care (68% lower) when compared to a similar group of patients who did not receive the intervention. Intervention group patients were also 78% less likely to be admitted to a nursing home. These patients also evidenced significant improvements in several measures of quality of life and functional status.

The CCCS experience is comparable to the outcomes noted by Resource Link of Iowa. To establish the efficacy of these approaches, a randomized controlled trial comparing telephone and videophone care for follow-up care of veterans with heart failure is currently being conducted at the Iowa City VA Medical Center. This 4-year study will evaluate the efficacy and cost-effectiveness of these technologies in reducing hospital admissions and improving symptom management and quality of life.

If You Build It, Will They Come?

Many investigators active in telehealth research and development have experienced the failure or slow adoption of technically excellent projects due to an apparent mismatch between the availability of new technologies and the readiness of the targeted user group. This defines the difference between vision and hallucination. Given the demographic realities of Iowa (and rural states like it), which include large numbers of elderly, poor, and geographically isolated citizens, a major component of the CIEH project focused on the readiness of potential users to participate in a health network. Studies included a gap analysis derived from county needs assessments, focus groups of healthcare providers and patients, and a statewide telephone survey involving a representative sample of 600 randomly selected Iowans.

Pertinent findings included the following:

- The underserved populations in Iowa include the elderly, women with children, and non-English-speaking persons—findings that were not revealed by the respondents in the statewide survey.
- Major barriers to healthcare access include limited transportation for the elderly and absence of specialists, particularly pediatric and OB/GYN physicians.
- Focus groups revealed wide variation in perceived healthcare needs and comfort with technology.
- Surprisingly high levels of satisfaction with available healthcare resources were revealed in the statewide survey. While we lack empirical data to identify causation, we speculate that cultural and social factors are at work.
- Respondents were found to be more technologically engaged and receptive than much of the literature in the area suggests, and more receptive to the idea of the CIEH than had been hypothesized.

These findings are encouraging, but only to a point. While the comfort level with technology is higher than anticipated, the underserved constitute a diverse collection of subgroups, and the remainder may not perceive the need for alternative approaches to care delivery. These types of studies need to be repeated in additional rural and urban settings in order to be of general usefulness.

Conclusion

Access to health care is an important, though not singular, determinant of health status for individuals and populations. In rural and some urban settings, the physical access to health care is limited by distance to, or relative scarcity of, healthcare providers. The potential to mediate inadequate access using technology has been often cited as a primary driving force for the development of telehealth. Unfortunately, the widespread implementation of telehealth has not occurred to date, for a number of reasons.

At the same time, several major trends have emerged that may inform future visions of health care. The first of these includes the rapid development and spread of the Internet, connected computers, and users, such that as many as half of U.S. citizens use the Internet on some basis. The second trend has been present for at least two decades in this country. The site of healthcare delivery has been migrating at an increasing rate from hospital to outpatient clinic to patient home. The U.S. demographics suggest that this trend will continue indefinitely. The intersection of these two trends would be the use of the Internet to meet various healthcare needs. Indeed, much of this is ongoing today, with many individuals using the Internet, and particularly the World Wide Web, to communicate health questions and concerns and obtain information. In many respects, this trend has already had a significant impact on healthcare delivery and provider-patient interactions.

There is a flip side to the technology revolution, as it pertains to health care. If half of Americans are using the Internet to improve their health and finding it useful, what about the half that currently do not access the Internet for whatever reason? Is it possible that this nonparticipative half might actually constitute a group in which the need for access to information and services is greater than the half already online? This is highly likely, as the unconnected group historically is older, less affluent, and more remote. So, as a society, this presents a basic problem. If access to online resources is beneficial, the optimal benefit will only be achievable if there is widespread, ubiquitous connectivity to the population. Is such a thing even possible? And under what circumstances would it occur? It is possible that universal access to the Internet might be achieved over time through "market forces"—price and availability on a par with the telephone or television. However, the adoption of simple Internet appliances and high-speed Internet connectivity has been slow and disappointing. Even if near-universal access could be established for a population, is it likely that a rational network for healthcare delivery purposes will emerge? It is unlikely without public health and planning carried out at a population level.

Acknowledgments. This work is supported in part by grant N01-LM-6-3548 from the National Library of Medicine and a VA HSR&D Career Development award to B.J.W.

References

1. Balas EA, Jaffrey R, Kuperman GJ, et al. Electronic communication with patients: evaluation of distance medicine technology. JAMA 1997;278:152–159.
2. Mair F, Whitten P. Systematic review of studies of patient satisfaction with telemedicine. BMJ 2000;320:1517–1520.
3. Currell R, Urquhart C, Wainwright P, Lewis R. Telemedicine versus face to face patient care: effects on professional practice and health care outcomes (Cochrane Review). In: Cochrane Library, issue 4. Oxford: Update Software, 2001.
4. Hersh W, Helfand M, Wallace J, et al. Clinical outcomes resulting from telemedicine interventions: a systematic review. BMC Medical Informatics and Decision Making 2001;1(5).
5. Berland GK, Elliott MN, Morales LS, et al. Health information on the Internet: accessibility, quality, and readability in English and Spanish. JAMA 2001;285:2612–2621.
6. D'Alessandro DM, Kingsley P, Johnson-West J. The readability of pediatric patient education materials on the World Wide Web. Arch Pediatr Adolesc Med 2001;155:807–812.
7. Hoffman-Goetz L, Clarke JN. Quality of breast cancer sites on the World Wide Web. Can J Public Health 2000;91:281–284.
8. D'Alessandro MP, Galvin JR, Colbert SI, et al. Solutions to challenges facing a university digital library and press. J Am Med Informatics Assoc 2000;246–253.
9. The Diabetes Control and Complications Trial (DCCT) Research Group. The effect of intensive treatment of diabetes in the development and progression of long-term complications in insulin-dependent diabetes mellitus. N Engl J Med 1993;329:977–986.
10. American Diabetes Association (ADA). Standards of medical care for patients with diabetes mellitus. Diabetes Care 2000;23(suppl 1):S32-S42. Available at http://www.biomedcentral.com/1472-6947/1/5.
11. Chin T. Some California physicians will be paid for online advice. Available at http://www.ama-assn.org/sci-pubs/amnews/pick_02/bisb1125.htm, 2002.
12. Miller TE, Derse AR. Between strangers: the practice of medicine online. Health Affairs 2002;21:168–179.
13. Relay Health. Relay Health webVisit study results. Available at http://www.relayhealth.com/rh/general/aboutUs/studyResults.aspx.
14. Kemper P, Murtaugh CM. Lifetime use of nursing home care. N Engl J Med 1991;324:595600.
15. Gardner S, Frantz R, Specht J, et al. How accurate are chronic wound assessments using interactive video technology? J Gerontol Nurs 2001;27(1):15–20.
16. Specht J, Wakefield B, Flanagan J. Evaluating the cost of one telehealth application connecting an acute and long term care setting. J Gerontol Nurs 2001;27(1):34–39.
17. Johnson-Mekota J, Maas M, Buresh K, et al. A nursing application of telecommunications: measurement of satisfaction for patients and providers. J Gerontol Nurs 2001;27(1):28–33.
18. Meyer M, Kobb R, Ryan P. Virtually healthy: chronic disease management in the home. J Dis Manag 2002;5(2):87–94.

Section II
Research and Development

II
Introduction: The Impact of the Internet on the Healthcare Consumer's Knowledge Development

EDWARD D. MARTIN

The communication of information and the acquisition of knowledge are, and have been for centuries, a cornerstone of our social and economic evolution. In ancient times icons and magnificent hand-painted, handwritten parchment scrolls were known to only the learned and scholarly. Knowledge resided at a few great cities and was passed on through generations by only a cadre of scholars. Gutenberg's printing press and movable type exploded the reach of the written word. Linotype and the word processor with direct connection to the printer's plate flashed printed media overnight throughout the world.

Undoubtedly, the Internet and Web technology created a most curious change. The concept of the "forward push" of information into published, printed works made available to consumers through libraries and book stores was remarkably transformed into an "outward push" of information into a global knowledge space, enabling the individual to *pull* information from anywhere in the world at any time of day or night. The Internet has brought about profound changes in how we communicate and how we acquire knowledge, and will become one of those great discoveries or inventions that we take for granted. In the next three chapters, Dixie B. Baker, Ph.D., and Daniel Masys, M.D.; John S. Parker, M.D.; and a collaboration of Ron D. Appel, Ph.D., and Celia Boyer discuss the Internet's impact on health care in a discussion that takes the reader from concept to extraordinary application.

Baker and Masys present an intriguing chapter on the technical architecture of the first research system built to enable consumers to view their own health information within a secure and private Web environment. They present details regarding this significant scientific work, including a description of the technical architecture of the PCASSO system and the study's results. With sufficient security protections in place, consumers feel confident that they can send healthcare transactions over the Internet architecture and that their privacy will be protected; an impact that could have dramatic consequences for healthcare information exchange between providers and patients.

Parker, in his usual way, takes the stark reality of little or no interface to the medical system via the Internet to the most extraordinary lengths. He explores the possibility of do-it-yourself health care aided by a browser, and challenges the reader to see beyond the status quo in healthcare delivery and provider–insurer–patient interaction. Do-it-yourself health care would be facilitated by medical knowledge acquired and directly applied by exercising consumer power over the Internet.

Appel and Boyer bring the questions of reliability and credibility of healthcare information into focus. Healthcare consumers are making personal, sometimes life-altering, decisions based on information they find online. Appel and Boyer explore the delicate task of finding a balance between the Internet as a free flow of information and the scientific validity of the information presented.

There is no question that the Internet is a vehicle for change now and into the future. It will cause change in medicine as it has caused change in other businesses that depend on the forces of the market. The effects of the Internet on medicine will be slower by comparison than those on other traditional markets because of the dictum in medicine to "do no harm" to the patient. In designing Internet-based systems that will be delivering healthcare information and knowledge to users, we must think of those users as potential patients and give them the same considerations with respect to safety and personal privacy that they receive from their family physician. That means that we must consider it our responsibility to ensure that the systems we build protect individual privacy and "do no harm."

Consumers expect change, and they want to be able to interact with their healthcare provider and their healthcare system as they do with their stockbroker or their favorite merchants on the Web. Privacy, the credibility of medical information, and the ability to correctly use that information for decision making will be essential features of the medical Internet. We must create the environment for consumers to feel at least as secure as they do when transacting business or viewing information from stockbrokers, mortgage lenders, and educational institutions. The medical consumer is a vital part of the supply-and-demand system that drives the world economy today and into the future. We cannot afford to fail to meet the medical consumers' needs and to empower them to assume a greater role in their care. We need to carefully identify the best approach to these challenges and act on them professionally and responsibly. The Internet will have an impact on how health is maintained and how care is delivered. The authors of the chapters in this section suggest we are at a crossroads in health care, and we must be careful to effectively and responsibly use the tools that are available to improve consumer access, understanding, and quality of life.

5
PCASSO: Vanguard in Patient Empowerment

DIXIE B. BAKER AND DANIEL MASYS

In 1996 the National Library of Medicine (NLM) funded a research project called Patient Centered Access to Secure Systems Online (PCASSO), which was proposed by Science Applications International Corporation (SAIC) in collaboration with the University of California, San Diego (UCSD). The project was designed to apply state-of-the-art security to the communication of clinical information over the Internet. At the project's inception, several prototype Web-based clinical information systems existed,[1-5] but all were explicitly designed for the benefit of health professionals—to enable them to view patient information stored on an enterprise server protected by a "firewall." Further, most early Internet experiments simply attempted to duplicate existing care models and lines of communication using the new medium. The concept of enabling patients to view their own complete medical record over the Internet was considered by the liberal-minded as radical and by the traditionalists as completely insane. PCASSO was conceived with the premise that the full potential of the ubiquitous Internet lies in its potential to enable new channels of communication between providers and patients, and to empower patients with the knowledge they need to participate actively in their own care.

The PCASSO project applied high-assurance methodologies and technologies originally developed by the Department of Defense, as well as standard World Wide Web technologies, to enable the search and retrieval of identifiable health information, including patient demographics, medications, lab tests, and transcription reports. The PCASSO model enforced a role-based security policy in which each user was granted only those accesses and privileges necessary to perform the activities associated with that user's role. The project was groundbreaking within the healthcare industry from two perspectives. First, it was the first project that allowed patients to view their entire medical records, and the audit of accesses to those records, over the Internet—thus breaking new ground in patient empowerment. Second, it was the first (and, to date, only) project to apply high-assurance methods and technologies, such as label-based access control, to the healthcare domain. As such, the PCASSO project has attracted the interest of the healthcare industry worldwide.[6-8] At the 1997 annual Symposium of the American Medical Informatics Association (AMIA), PCASSO was presented the Priscilla Mayden Award as the best "new model of or approach to improving information flow or knowledge management, and experimental observations documenting the successful implementation of the model." By the end of the project, PCASSO had gained broad recognition as a vanguard in patient empowerment and robust security architecture for Internet access.[9,10]

The PCASSO Model

The PCASSO team adopted a security policy that explicitly recognized the rights and responsibilities of providers and their patients, and the potentially hostile environment that is the Internet. The PCASSO model enforced its security policy through a multifactor user authentication strategy, a role-based access-control scheme, and accountability provisions that attributed all system actions to the users who initiated them. Technical details relating to the security model and concept of operations,[11] the system architecture and design,[12] the approach for dealing with client-side vulnerabilities,[8,13,14] and the high-assurance methodologies and technologies employed[14] have been described elsewhere. Sufficient for our purposes here is to describe the PCASSO model as a "high-assurance" application server that served a single application—one that enabled the user to view a patient's electronic medical record through a standard Web browser. By "high-assurance," we are referring to the fact that the methodologies and technologies used in specifying, designing, building, and operating the model were based on those previously prescribed and used to build systems that handle classified information.[15,16] These methods are far more stringent, and the technologies much stronger, than those used by typical "e-commerce" applications. Our requirement for high assurance was driven by the fact that the PCASSO system did not sanitize or filter out any data. So "deniable" data[17] such as genetic, HIV/AIDS, mental health, substance abuse, and sexually transmitted disease information were stored in the PCASSO clinical data repository (CDR) and made available for viewing over the Internet. Our reasoning was that information whose unauthorized disclosure could cause permanent and irrevocable damage to an individual's insurability, employability, and standard of living is at least as worthy of protection as information whose unauthorized disclosure could "reasonably be expected to cause serious damage to the national security."[18]

To establish the context for our discussion here, we describe the PCASSO model from the perspective of the consumer experience. To obtain a PCASSO account required that users be at least 18 years of age and active UCSD patients; that they have a personal computer and Internet access; and that they be authorized by their primary care provider, after signing the informed-consent document. At the time of registration, users were given a user guide; a password; a diskette containing their unique public-key certificate; and a

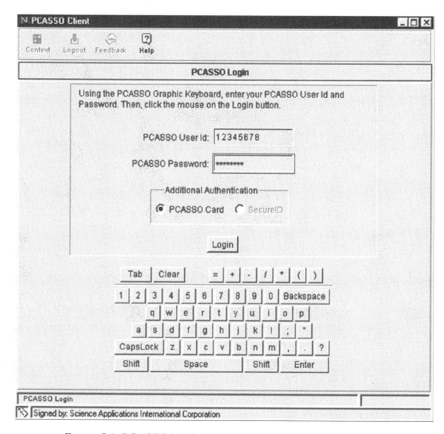

FIGURE 5.1. PCASSO log-in screen. (Reprinted with permission.)

"PCASSO card," a laminated card containing a set of random numbers that were synchronized with a corresponding list stored on the server. [a] After logging into their preferred Internet service provider, the users would point the Web browser (Netscape Navigator or Microsoft Internet Explorer) to the PCASSO server by entering PCASSO's URL, which for our evaluation was http://medicine.ucsd.edu/pcasso, where users were given the option to log on as registered users. The PCASSO server then downloaded to the user's computer a small software application (Java client applet) that displayed the login screen shown in Figure 5.1.

    User authentication was a multistep operation. To reduce risks inherent in a personal computer,[13] a graphical keyboard was used to enter all security-critical and patient-confidential information, such as users' passwords and

---

[a]The PCASSO team constrained its design options to mechanisms that would impose no additional cost on the patient above the cost of a personal computer and software, and Internet access. In a "real" implementation, one would want to consider other options, such as smart cards and challenge-response tokens.

patients' names. On the graphical keyboard, users entered their user ID and password. PCASSO then asked them to insert the read-only, encrypted diskette, which contained their private encryption key. Invisible to users, the client application and the server used their respective public-private key pairs to authenticate each other ("shaking hands"), after which the user was informed that a secure connection had been established. Note that this mutual "handshake" is different from what happens on most e-commerce sites, which typically use only server authentication to establish the encrypted link.

PCASSO then asked the users to input the next character string that appeared on their "PCASSO card." When the user entered the number the server expected, authentication was completed, and the demographics screen shown in Figure 5.2 was displayed. The tabs indicate the three types of information the patient could view: demographics, laboratory test results, and physician notes. In addition, by clicking on the Audit Log icon at the top of the screen, users could view a list of the individuals who had been granted the right to view their record, and a list of those individuals who had actually viewed the

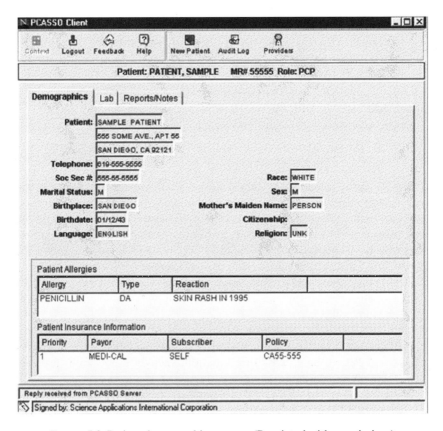

FIGURE 5.2. Patient demographics screen. (Reprinted with permission.)

record through the PCASSO system. When users were finished, they could log out using the Logout icon at the top of the screen. Alternatively, after a 10-minute period of inactivity, PCASSO automatically terminated the session.

Benefits and Challenges in Patient Empowerment

Involving patients in the provision of their own care offers enormous benefits to both the patients and their providers. Physicians recognize that the patient is their primary source of information regarding symptoms and perceived reactions to treatment. They would further assert that the critical factor in the effectiveness of treatments is the patient's compliance with prescribed protocols. So patients already are involved in their own care. "Empowering" patients simply acknowledges their shared responsibility and builds upon the trust that has historically served as the foundation of the provider-patient relationship. The empowerment comes from giving patients greater access to information and from facilitated patient-provider communications. Empowered patients are better equipped to manage their own health, to educate themselves regarding their health condition, and to play an active part in their treatment.

Along with the benefits come a number of challenges, the greatest of which may be achieving the cultural changes required to achieve a consumer-focused, service-delivery system.[9] These cultural challenges pose several risks that were reflected in the concerns of UCSD's Institutional Review Board (IRB) when it reviewed PCASSO's evaluation plan and approved the use of human subjects for the evaluation phase of the project.[19] Identified risks included the following:

1. The risk of unauthorized access outside the provider's span of control;
2. The risk that the consumer may receive and act upon misunderstood, confusing, or potentially erroneous information; and
3. The risk that physicians may hold back or distort their recorded information in response to concerns over the patient's seeing it.

The first risk—that unauthorized individuals may obtain access to private patient information—was the primary motivation for the PCASSO research. The Internet offers a convenient and cost-effective means of supporting patient-centered health care. It delivers an abundance of information; it has spawned virtual communities that span the globe; and its ability to support one-to-one communications from anywhere is ideally suited to support patient-provider communications. Unfortunately, the Internet was constructed using technologies specifically designed for "open" communications, and the Internet protocol (IP) provides no protection for confidential information. Further, technologies the Internet has spawned have introduced new vulnerabilities.[20] The PCASSO project sought to address known vulnerabilities in the client PC, in the communications link, and in the server.

The IRB seemed confident that the PCASSO model had implemented measures to counter the Internet risks, but IRB members were concerned that since the patient would be using the PCASSO system in the home, another family member or visitor might accidentally or purposely view that patient's private health information. The team responded by describing our method of physically validating the user's identity at the time of registration and PCASSO's strong, multifactor authentication scheme involving a password, a private key, and a challenge-response token (the PCASSO card). For a family member to be able to log in using a legitimate user's identity, that individual not only would need to know the user's user ID and password, but also would have to gain possession of the diskette and PCASSO card associated with that account, and would need to understand the PCASSO log-in process. With respect to inadvertent or intentional reading of private data from a PCASSO screen, the user's guide distributed at registration set forth the users' responsibilities in providing the physical protection necessary to keep their information private. Finally, the client design contained several features that prevented other PC users and malicious code running on the client from capturing the user's health data—the print and write-to-disk capabilities were disabled, and memory was cleared of text representations of the patient's name.

The second risk—that patients may receive and act upon misunderstood, confusing, or even erroneous information—is a significant risk inherent in the use of the Internet as a source of medical information. The Internet has been characterized as "a medium in which anyone with a computer can serve simultaneously as author, editor, and publisher and can fill any or all of these roles anonymously if he or she so chooses."[21] Because users can post anything they want, the Internet inevitably contains a great deal of inaccurate and misleading information. As a result, the traditional peer-review process for medical guidance is effectively circumvented. The IRB's concern in this area related to the fact that a patient potentially could see a lab result or dictated note before the physician had seen that information. This risk existed because information was sent to the PCASSO server as it became available, rather than being reviewed or prefiltered, so that information was available to patients and providers simultaneously. The concern was the possibility that psychological harm could result if the patient were to see surprising, confusing, or puzzling information before the provider had had a chance to explain it. For example, what would happen if a patient saw a new diagnosis of a disease such as cancer before the physician had had a chance to prepare the patient and explain the diagnosis?

An analysis of this "out-of-the-blue" diagnosis scenario[18] showed that a definitive diagnosis nearly always follows a specific test or procedure the provider has ordered, rather than a general screening test. For example, cancer requires a tissue biopsy and a procedure to obtain that tissue. Any diagnostic procedure requires the patient's informed consent, which most certainly will include an explanation of the procedure and the potential outcomes. Nonetheless, the PCASSO project acknowledged that in a "real" implementation, one would want to provide supplementary, authoritative information resources to help patients understand what they read in their record. So the PCASSO project incorporated several safeguards, including filtering out "pending" results so that only "final" results were stored in the CDR; warning language in the informed-consent document; a toll-free "hotline" and formal triage capability; and IRB involvement in handling any adverse effects of "information toxicity."[18]

The third risk—that giving patients access to their own health information might diminish the value of physicians' notes—reflects the asymmetry of power that exists in physician-patient relationships. Some physicians record candid and detailed observations so long as they know that only peers, and not patients, will see their notes. The fallacy in this thinking is that even in PCASSO's early days, patients had the right to request a copy of their information at any time in most states. The Privacy Regulation promulgated pursuant to the Health Insurance Portability and Accountability Act (HIPAA) extends this right to all 50 states.[22] However, PCASSO used a label-based access control mechanism to enable primary care providers to specifically label data within the PCASSO CDR "patient deniable," which blocked the patient from viewing the data through the PCASSO interface. Also, the import function enforced rules for applying sensitivity labels as the data were loaded into the CDR. For example, one rule implemented in the PCASSO model was that all notes originating in the psychiatry department were labeled "patient deniable" by default.

As part of its due diligence, the IRB asked the general counsel for the University of California system to review the project plan for potential risks to the institution. The general counsel concluded that the potential benefits associated with the project far outweighed the risks. In fact, the advisors saw greatest risk in *not* providing patients access to their own information. They further noted that PCASSO offered the potential to reduce UCSD's liability by virtually ensuring that results would be reviewed expeditiously by someone—be it patient or provider.

Results and Observations

In 2000 a Harris survey of 1000 consumers 18 years of age or over revealed the following[23]:

- 89% would use a nurse triage service to help them manage a chronic medical condition, and they would like this service to be available via the phone and the Internet.
- 40% expressed frustration at having to see their physicians in person to get answers to simple healthcare questions.
- 83% wanted their lab tests to be available online.
- 69% wanted online charts for monitoring chronic conditions. Consumers also thought their doctors should use automated systems to help them better manage their care.

- 84% wanted their doctors to send them electronic alerts (e.g., time for a flu shot).
- 80% wanted to receive personalized medical information online from their physician following an office visit.

The results from our research essentially reinforced this study's findings. The consumers who participated in the PCASSO study expressed appreciation for the ability to view their health information online, frustration with their lack of control over their own health, and a desire to communicate with their providers electronically. Complete and detailed results are discussed elsewhere.[19] Here we focus on results directly related to patient empowerment.

The evaluation criteria for the PCASSO system corresponded to those used by the Food and Drug Administration to evaluate potential pharmaceuticals: Is it safe, and is it effective? Over the 6-month patient evaluation period, 41 patients were registered as PCASSO users, and 26 (63%) actually used the PCASSO system one or more times. At the end of each use, the user was asked to complete a feedback form addressing several areas: reasonableness of the security features, ease of use, usefulness of the data, and system effectiveness.

As shown in Figure 5.3, the consumers' perceptions of what was reasonable and appropriate for protecting their health information was somewhat different from the perceptions of providers. Every patient who responded to our questions regarding the reasonableness and appropriateness of PCASSO's security features rated them very satisfactory. The contrast between the opinions of our consumers and our providers was greater with respect to ease of use (Fig. 5.4). Our patients did not find the PCASSO system particularly difficult to use, regardless of their perceived level of comfort with computers and the Internet. Even those users who judged their computer skills "fair" or "novice" rated the PCASSO system either "somewhat easy" or "very easy" to

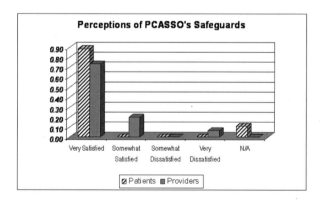

Figure 5.3. Reasonableness and appropriateness of PCASSO's safeguards.

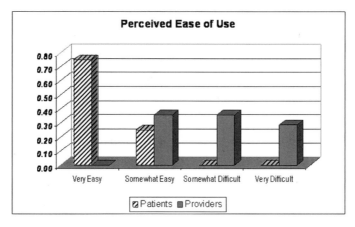

FIGURE 5.4. Perceived ease of use.

use. One might speculate that patients perceived any inconvenience in using the system as an acceptable side effect of the "safeguards" they desired. Another relevant point is that for patients, PCASSO was the first and only means through which the patients could view their health information electronically, while the physicians could view the data much more easily through UCSD's internal clinical system.

As shown in Figure 5.5, all of the patients who provided feedback judged the value of having access to their medical records as either "somewhat valuable" or "very valuable," and the candid comments the patients offered rein-

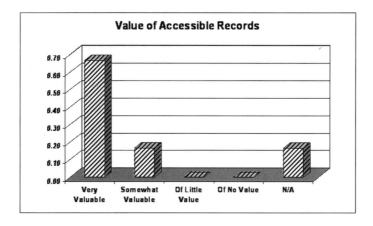

FIGURE 5.5. Value of accessibility to records to patients.

forced this opinion. Many comments expressed gratitude to the project for enabling patients to view their own information and frustration with the lack of control over their own health:

- "Thank you for this 'peek' into our own medical records. So often patients seem to feel at the mercy of the HMOs and at least this may alleviate some of that distrust."
- "I was at the lab this morning and some results are posted already....Very impressed!!"
- "It was great to be able to read my lab results as my physician has not reported them to me."
- "As one who has always been involved in my healthcare decisions, I value that I have access to this information."
- "Great system, I find it very user-friendly and feel very confident that my privacy is maintained at all times."

A number of comments were questions and observations reflecting known effects that were not adequately explained to the patients. For example, several patients commented that some of their lab results were not available—an effect resulting from our decision to preload the CDR with only the most recent additions to patient records. Another patient observed that two of the three individuals identified as his primary care providers were actually specialists—an effect resulting from a loader rule we implemented that automatically assigned the primary-care-provider role to any physician whose name appeared on a procedure order received in an HL7 message.

Other comments were explicit questions about what the patient could expect to see in the system:

- "Will my primary care doctor's notes appear here, too?"
- "I am unclear about what information will be available here."
- "I opened the file, and there was no information in it. Why is that?"

These results reinforce the importance of providing clear and complete user guidance regarding how to use the system and what content the consumer should expect. In addition, some patients requested additional information or features, such as a key to the notations found in a lab report, and records of charges billed to an insurance company.

Perhaps the most valuable comments, and those most relevant to this discussion, are those that reflect how having access to their own medical information affected patients' attitudes and behavior. When asked on the feedback form whether the service and information PCASSO provided influenced the user's personal actions, the responses were equally distributed among "yes," "no," and "not yet." However, one individual commented that he had detected an error in the lab test that was conducted and that he had called the doctor's office to let the staff know that the lab test performed was different from the test the doctor was to have ordered. Another patient reported that because she knew that her lab results would be viewable through PCASSO when they were available, she had not felt the need to call her doctor's office. Several patients commented that they intended to discuss the contents of their record with their primary care provider. For example, one individual asked for the ability to print the record so he could take it with him for his next doctor's visit. Some patients said that after checking PCASSO and seeing that their lab results were not yet there, they had refrained from calling their doctors. So our data show that empowering patients with information is likely to reduce the need for certain types of calls to the doctor's office.

Although the PCASSO model provided no mechanism to communicate directly with the physician, several patients used the feedback form to do so:

- "I should have cytology results posted (done on July 20) as well as X-ray on July 27. Can you tell me when these might be posted? Thanks."
- "My address has changed."

These kinds of comments confirm the Harris finding that not only do consumers want to be able to see their health information, they also want the ability to communicate with their physicians electronically.

Conclusion

The PCASSO project was a true vanguard in patient empowerment. To this day, we know of no other project that enables patients to view their entire medical record over the Internet. Our results reinforce the notion that patients want access to their health information and that they expect a high level of security protection for it. Further, empowered patients are willing and able to respond appropriately as active participants in their own care.

Acknowledgment   The work reported here was supported by a Health Information Infrastructure research contract N01 LM63537-00 from the U.S. National Library of Medicine.

References

1. Cimino JJ, Socratous S, Clayton PD. Internet as clinical information system: application development using the World Wide Web. J Am Med Informatics Assoc 1995;2(5):273–283.
2. Chute CC, Crowson DL, Buntrock JD. Medical information retrieval and WWW browsers at Mayo. In: Gardner RM, ed. Proceedings of the 1995 annual symposium on computer applications in medical care, New Orleans, November 1995. 903–907.
3. Jagannathan V, Reddy YV, et al. An overview of the CERC ARTEMIS project. In: Gardner RM, ed. Proceedings of the 1995 annual symposium on computer applications in medical care, New Orleans, November 1995. 12–16.
4. Kahn CE, Bell DS. WebSTAR: platform-independent structured reporting using World-Wide Web technology. In: Hripcsak G, ed. Proceedings of the 1995 spring congress of AMIA, Boston, MA, June 1995. 86.

5. Masys DR, Baker DB. Patient-Centered Access to Secure Systems Online (PCASSO): a secure approach to clinical data access via the World Wide Web. J Am Med Informatics Assoc 1997;4(Fall Symposium Suppl):340–343.

6. Baker DB. PCASSO: ensuring patient confidentiality on the Internet. Presented at the Fourth International Multimedia to the Home Conference: Building on Bandwidth, Saskatoon, Saskatchewan, Canada, August 20, 1999.

7. New Zealand Health Information Services, "Health Links," http://www.nzhis.govt.nz/links.html, 2002.

8. Baker DB, Masys DR. PCASSO: a design for secure communication of personal health information via the Internet. Int J Med Informatics 1999;54:97–104.

9. Borzo G. PCASSO with a mouse. amednews.com, October 13, 1997, http://www.ama-assn.org/sci-pubs/amnews/net_97/logo1013.htm, 2002.

10. Tsai CC, Starren J. Patient participation in electronic medical records. Medical Student JAMA 2001;285:1765. Accessible online at http://www.ama-assn.org/sci-pubs/msjama/articles/vol_285/no_13/jms0404012.htm#5.

11. Masys DR, Baker DB, Barnhart R, Buss T. PCASSO: a secure architecture for access to clinical data via the Internet. In: Proceedings of the MEDINFO '98, International Medical Informatics Association, August 1998.

12. Baker D, Barnhart R, Buss T. PCASSO: applying and extending state-of-the-art security in the healthcare domain. In: Proceedings of the Annual Computer Security Applications Conference, San Diego, CA, December 1997.

13. Masys DR, Baker DB. Protecting clinical data on Web client computers: the PCASSO approach. J Am Med Informatics Assoc 1998;5(Fall Symposium Suppl):366–370.

14. Baker DB, Masys DR, Jones RL, Barnhart RM. Assurance: the power behind PCASSO security. J Am Med Informatics Assoc 1999;6(Fall Symposium Suppl):666-670. "Best paper" award nominee AMIA fall symposium.

15. U.S. Department of Defense, Department of Defense Trusted Computer System Evaluation Criteria, DoD 5200.28-STD, December 1985.

16. Common criteria for information technology security evaluation, Part 3: security assurance requirements, version 2.1, CCIMB-99-033, August 1999.

17. Dick RS, Steen EB, eds., Institute of Medicine. The computer-based patient record: an essential technology for health care. Washington, DC: National Academy Press, 1991.

18. Executive Order 12958—classified national security information. Federal Register, April 20, 1995;19826.

19. Masys D, Baker D, Butros A, Cowles KE. Giving patients access to their medical records: the PCASSO experience. J Am Med Informatics Assoc 2002;181–191.

20. Baker DB. Protecting life and health in the midst of electronic and Internet mayhem. Managed Care Interface 2000;13(6):81-87.

21. Fallis D. Inaccurate consumer health information on the Internet: criteria for evaluating potential solutions. Proceedings of the American Medical Informatics Association Annual Symposium, 1999.

22. Department of Health and Human Services. Standards for privacy of individually identifiable health information. Billing code 4150-04M. Federal Register, 45 CFR parts 160-164, December 28, 2000.

23. Consumers demand combination of "high-tech" and "high-touch" personalized services to manage healthcare needs. Harris Interactive, http://www.harrisinteractive.com, 2000.

6
Consumer Expectations Demand Client-Focused Technology: So Near, Yet So Far

JOHN S. PARKER

This chapter has been difficult for me to write. Originally, I planned to review the information technology available to the medical community from three distinct areas: (1) early research and development; (2) advanced technical research centers; and (3) technology that is in the early stages of use, but is still funded by research and development dollars. The goal was to excite you about things to come. The chapter looked like a list in prose format and said nothing about how the technology should be adopted into the medical community at large. There was a total absence of technology involving the client at the front end; in fact, the client, in my experience, is seldom the beneficiary. I procrastinated a lot and struggled. Frustrated, I asked what's missing and went on with another day.

It was a normal day. I sent and received about a hundred e-mails. I browsed and read several articles from the nation's leading newspapers online. I had multiple appointments and met many interesting people. By the miracle of a password, my bank account, stock portfolio, mortgage, and insurance information was checked to proclaim my wealth or lack thereof at this precise minute of the day. A few items were purchased on the Internet and a few bills were paid with instant notification of completion and a code to check the status later. I made an airline reservation and decided not to rent a car.

My mind was consumed with the pressing issues of the day. The Internet brought mountains of information from numerous sources. A few hours of study brought fusion and convergence of the data that I needed.

My health is important to me. I wanted to know what the trends were on my blood pressure, and some other medical data over the past year to verify that my medications and behavioral changes were making a difference. That couldn't be done at the moment. I would have to go home and search through the large paper file labeled medical information. If I found the correct information, I would then take time to set up a spreadsheet on the computer and try to fill in the blanks. One or two days later, if I worked at it, I might be able to graph something. It would have a lot of gaps. Most of the essential data (financial, stock portfolio, insurance policies, mortgage, credit card data, and banking) of my life is on someone's secure Web site, trended, and updated daily. Not my medical record, and it certainly wouldn't be supported with search engines and graphics to facilitate feedback and help influence my behavior in the future. Oh well… someday…maybe.

Technology and information has influenced the practice of medicine for decades. When you look at the focus of that influence, it remains in the areas of diagnosis and treatment or in the business area of medicine that enables the reimbursement for the use of the applied technology or services. If the medical business information technology is not directly related to the classic billable revenue stream or designed to improve capture of costs, it is hard to find in the medical system. It is a tough statement to make but we haven't connected the client to our system.

Change Is Difficult

Medicine is a classic supply and demand system. The simple principal driver of the system today is illness. The type of illness, the difficulty of diagnosis and the treatment drive the technology to be used. The patient's medical knowledge as a demand is starting to cause increasing pressure on the system. Our clients are asking for the use of cutting edge technology and drugs, for example. Payers are critical about the growing amount of public announcements of cutting-edge technologies and pharmaceutical and other advertising that usually ends with, "Ask your doctor about…" A knowledgeable, demanding consumer may be a nightmare for the payer, but may be the "undiscovered" driver to cost containment in the long run. Currently, managing the care or tailoring reimbursement controls demand.

Knowledge is a burden unless you can do something with it. We must have a system that allows people to use their knowledge directly if we want our educated clients to take care of themselves. However, there are two intermediaries: the medical profession itself and the payer. Individuals cannot leverage their knowledge directly. For example, they cannot get a laboratory test, treatment, or medication without entering the traditional system and paying the "middleman" a transit cost. That transit cost is expensive because it bears liability costs. Resistance to change is profoundly influenced by the classical approaches to reimbursement and liability.

Knowledge Is One of the Keys

If we are going to use technology to contain the cost of medical care, we need to engage the knowledgeable client on the front end of the system. People who must function within society drive the accumulation of knowledge for different reasons. Who you are and what you do is irrelevant. You must have specific knowledge to survive. The sophistication of that personal knowledge is related to its functional environment. Knowledge allows us to build on a known to solve an unknown. Knowledge allows us to deal with the environment. How we function, based on that knowledge, determines whether we survive or perish in a particular environment. Years ago, knowledge resided within specific persons, universities, or libraries. Now, sources of knowledge (information) are fully available, global in nature, and found throughout the world by the strike of a key on a computer. Today, you do not have to be "qualified" by some guild to have access to the knowledge.

The speed at which we accumulate knowledge is related to need or potential application. Knowledge gathered in a focused manner generally causes something to happen, especially if it improves one's environment or has a direct relationship to one's well-being or economic return. Specific knowledge at a specific time and place is mandatory as the complexities of our individual environments increase. Knowledge on demand is a key to good decision making, provided the substance and source of the knowledge is verified, certified, or authenticated in some way by some authority. If we accept the fact that credible medical knowledge can be provided to consumers by multiple technological methods (electronic, print, and voice) for specific medical conditions, don't you think there would be a reasonable expectation that consumers could use that information directly for their benefit without an intermediary?

What Are the Consumer's Expectations?

I am not sure we have asked the right question in the past. We ask consumers what kind of health care they want. We never get beyond the rudimentary answers of quality, access, and cost. We should rephrase the question by asking how they would interface with the healthcare system if it were like a bank, mortgage company, insurance company, wholesaler, or retailer that allowed access to information and provided services via a Web-based presentation layer. I suspect they would like to see us have an electronic medical record that they could read. They would like the ability to contact us, ask questions, get answers, make appointments, and then get therapeutics without having to physically enter the system. The bottom line here is that we have probably missed an opportunity by not asking the right question. Are we afraid to ask because our behavior would have to change, or because we would have to wrestle the issue of who is control of health care¾the provider or the consumer? Introducing this aspect of informatics and technology into medicine could change the behavior, liability, and reimbursement equilibrium of the system.

The Way Forward

Engaging the client is a critical behavioral move. A major healthcare system that is recognized for excellence in management and quality of care should consider convening a facilitated, small group of preselected educated consumers. The agenda should pose well-constructed critical questions to the group that creates a discussion that would surface possible attributes of a client-focused medical information system. Initial briefings could set the stage by describing other interactive systems seen today in the banking, finance, and insurance industries. The results of the session would be carefully reviewed, ideas selected, and a scalable pilot put into place.

[1]The Future

Available technology exceeds most of the needs to make dramatic improvements in the healthcare system today. We haven't put clients (patients) in control of how they spend their dollars in the system. Some would say we have, and that I just don't understand who the customers are today. The fact that it is *their* money is lost on our individual client because most financial transactions are between payer and provider¾neither being the recipient of the services directly. The consumers never feel that they have engaged in a business transaction¾services rendered, services paid for. It's invisible to them most of the time. In a situation like that it is easy to say or think that it is someone else's responsibility to decide whether or not I got what they paid for. That has to change. We must put the responsibility for judging and paying for services on the client in certain specified circumstances.

The combination of using medical knowledge, combined with an ability to purchase goods and services, in certain medical situations may be an interesting pilot project. Individuals could use their knowledge, assisted by appropriate, well-tested process mapping constructs, to purchase laboratory tests, use other diagnostics, arrive at a diagnosis, and then purchase the treatment directly. They may have access to advisory personnel or not. This could be a closely monitored pilot to see how consumers behave in a relatively free market. All of the transactions could be monitored instantaneously by watching their behavior on the front end, their purchases by electronic card, and outcomes measured. It would be interesting to see what segment of society could be given this freedom and whether it would be cost-effective. We could watch how the consumers used various levels of medical consultation for a fee versus open knowledge sources to solve their medical problems. We may learn that there is a domain of prehospitalization health care within which the consumer can function without entering the traditional healthcare system. Do we trust people to do "do-it-yourself" health care? People do their own plumbing, electrical work, and home construction¾why not some aspects of health care enabled by information technology?

Conclusion

This has been a glimpse into the possible uses of information technology in medicine. It involves the clients as direct customers and gives them empowerment to see their data, and proposes further liberation of the clients to be consumers online. If we constantly apply technology to the traditional practice, delivery pattern, and management, we may never see the real dynamics of technology, knowledge, business, and medicine and their effect on the cost of care in the future.

7
Steps Toward Reliable Online Consumer Health Information

RON D. APPEL AND CELIA BOYER

The latest advances in information technologies have allowed for the development of applications that have had tremendous repercussions in the healthcare field. Along with access, means must be provided to ensure that information is trustworthy and relevant. Certification of information quality can remain voluntary, preserving citizens' rights and promoting diversity. Collaboration among all Internet stakeholders is crucial to reducing conflicts of interest and for cost-effective distribution of quality health and medical information.

This chapter examines some of the problems arising from unprecedented access to vast quantities of health information made possible by the Internet. The role of search engines is explored and some of their associated problems are mentioned. We look at some of the policy initiatives that have been introduced in an effort to protect Internet citizens ("netizens") from exposure to information of highly variable quality. The most mature of these initiatives, the HONcode, is discussed in detail, along with new technologies capable of analyzing online health content also being developed by the Health on the Net Foundation. Finally, tentative conclusions are offered in the form of questions: as the Internet eludes regulation, as technologies and business models are introduced and superseded in ever-shorter cycles, how can we effectively deal with the new threats posed by information misuse?

Healthcare Information

Information, possibly the most valuable asset of a global society, seems to have a life of its own. Once limited to oral transmission, then by papyrus, movable type, and now the Internet, information is bound up with human progress, yet we are vulnerable to its misuse. Like a virus, it can quickly multiply out of control, it is difficult if not impossible to eliminate, and it can only be managed with varying degrees of success. Though information has become essential for the maintenance of health, it can take dangerous forms that must be addressed if they are not to cause harm.

A highly educated and well-informed public now demands better and more complete access to information. The number of citizens using the Internet to seek health information increases with each passing day, and health and medical information is being published online at an ever-increasing rate. For Internet users, the Web may now be their principal source of factual information, leaving television and other media to provide for their entertainment needs.

No longer must we call the research desk of our public library; consumers find themselves newly empowered to research their medical condition as they would their stock portfolio, and they can just as easily fall prey to misleading advice. Problems associated with mass media now play out in the online space: commercial interests clash with those of simplicity and common sense, and medical controversies continue to rage. Consumers are faced with a baffling array of information options, yet, despite our worst fears, little evidence points to the Internet as a source of mortal danger. Yet, while studies claim that consumers are satisfied with the quality of information they find, we cannot allow ourselves to become complacent when we understand the risks.

Official attempts to regulate online content cannot hope to keep pace with the developments of the medium, and may fall afoul of civil liberties protections. Indeed, it appears futile, not to say retrograde, to try to restrict the flow of online information. Yet, as Internet use becomes pervasive, something must be done to help users sort through an increasing and often contradictory mass of information.

To realize the potential of the Internet as a source of valuable healthcare information for the general public, patients, and practitioners, it is imperative to establish a validation system and standards of quality. International cooperation is needed for the establishment of standards, such as those governing the publication of medical literature.

Codes and Seals

Behavioral codes and means of evaluating information could provide useful criteria for medical/health Web sites that aspire to minimal ethical and quality standards. There are several initiatives at the global level, of which the most widely known and recognized is the Health on the Net Foundation (HON) (www.hon.ch) and its HONcode.

Of course, one cannot take into account everything published on the Internet because one of its main features is precisely the heterogeneity of its contents—reliable information along with unreliable information. So the benefit obtained is enormous, as is the harm done by spreading information without any kind of scientific validation.

Yet it is the nature of the Internet to resist attempts at institutionalization or ownership. Major players emerge and household names disappear overnight. Consumers demand autonomy, but seek validation. We must gain their trust even as we awaken their critical sense.

The first attempt at "truth in labeling" for online health content was the HONcode, brainchild of Prof. Jean-Raoul Scherrer of the Geneva University Hospitals. Introduced in 1996, the HONcode sets out eight principles for Web publishers, which, if followed, give the Web master the right to display HON's "seal of approval." The HONcode makes no attempt to judge the content of a medical/health Web site; however, the principles require Web publishers to disclose potential conflicts of interest, to attribute authorship to information sources, and to pledge to apply strict guidelines for the confidential treatment of users' personal information. A site should not only comply with the HONcode principles but also demonstrate how each principle is implemented.

Establishing trust is crucial in any relationship between a patient and a provider of health services. This applies not only to doctors and other caregivers, but also to information providers. If, previously, one could infer some level of trustworthiness from the context in which information appeared (bookstore, television network, lecture hall), this is no longer the case with the Internet. Any computer connected to the Web can deliver information, limited only by the technical means of its owner. Search engines rapidly discover any new sources but are not programmed to analyze the meaning of content they find. For a variety of obscure reasons, false or misleading information may appear at the top of a list of search results, competing with reliable, but less attractively packaged content.

With "information overload," the role of the healthcare professional as a teacher and advisor cannot be overlooked, strengthened by his or her role as a trusted intermediary between different users. Users choose the online healthcare information they think is reliable.

Furthermore, ethical codes are hard for users to understand. The "HONpatient" project will educate consumers to look for the HONcode seal and other reliability criteria while surfing the Web. Guidelines for Web masters are also being issued in an effort to educate online publishers to improve the quality of their Web sites and prepare them for accreditation.

Display of the HONcode seal marks information as meeting essential standards for online publishing of health and medical content. The HONcode seeks to create a "confidence space," where trustworthy information is easy to access and users are free to move among information sources without limits on their autonomy. At the same time, the disclosures and other assertions demanded of Web masters by the HONcode remind users of the need for a critical approach as they access health resources online.

Its simplicity and tolerance of diversity have earned the HONcode wide acceptance. However, for accreditation schemes such as the HONcode to fully succeed, effective public communication is needed to differentiate, in the minds of consumers and Web masters alike, the meaning of accreditation compared with that of specious awards or pay-for-placement listing schemes. The HONcode seal, displayed on the home page of accredited Web sites, links back to HON, enabling information searchers to learn more about the accreditation criteria (Fig. 7.1).

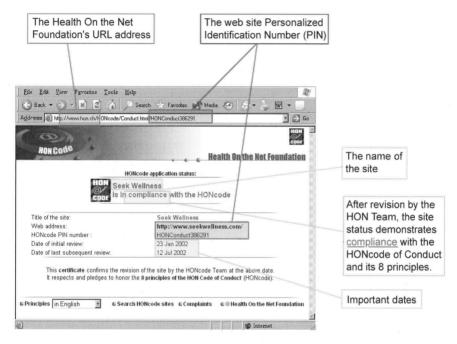

FIGURE 7.1. HONcode valid and official HONcode certificate. (Reprinted with permission.)

The HONcode is a voluntary program. Web publishers pledge to exceed the requirements stated in the principles. They contact HON not to obtain a rating or award, but to join a community sharing common principles. During the initial application process, Web masters are made aware of their site's possible short-comings and are urged to make changes to bring it into conformity. But the service performed by HON for health information professionals is also didactic. It has often been said that the goal of HON's application process is the ongoing education of the Web publisher, with accreditation as the reward. Even a site seriously lacking in the reliability criteria defined by HON can be brought into compliance through the application process itself.

Once admitted into the "confidence space" of HONcode accreditation, the Web master is expected to continue following the code of conduct as new content is added to the site. Periodic reevaluation of the site is part of the accreditation contract, and a site is subject to review at any time. Members of the community of accredited sites as well as the public are requested to be vigilant and report noncompliant sites to HON for follow-up. Accreditation may be suspended in cases of serious or repeated violations of the code.

The HONcode is a first step toward qualifying information as trustworthy based on the willingness of publishers to comply with an easy-to-follow set of ethical standards. How then are we to address the really difficult issue of the content itself? Peer review of the massive number of available documents is not reasonable; automation must be used to perform the validation function.

HONcode: The Principles

HONcode includes eight principles whose three key pillars are (1) identification of the site editors and their competencies, (2) citation of references to external sources, and (3) a clear distinction between advertising and scientific editorials.

The HONcode was initially and simultaneously written in English and French. As of November 2002, the HONcode is available in 23 languages: Arabic, Catalan, Chinese, Danish, Dutch, English, Finnish, French, German, Greek, Hungarian, Icelandic, Italian, Japanese, Korean, Malaysian, Norwegian, Polish, Portuguese, Russian, Spanish, Swedish, and Turkish. Following is the English version of the HONcode:

1. Authority: Any medical or health advice provided and hosted on this site will be given only by medically trained and qualified professionals unless a clear statement is made that a piece of advice offered is from a nonmedically qualified individual or organization.
2. Complementarity: The information provided on this site is designed to support, not replace, the relationship that exists between a patient/site visitor and his/her existing physician.
3. Confidentiality: Confidentiality of data relating to individual patients and visitors to a medical/health Web site, including their identity, is respected by this Web site. The Web site owners undertake to honor or exceed the legal requirements of medical/health information privacy that apply in the country and state where the Web site and mirror sites are located.
4. Attribution: Where appropriate, information contained on this site will be supported by clear references to source data and, where possible, have specific HTML links to that data. The date when a clinical page was last modified will be clearly displayed (e.g., at the bottom of the page).
5. Justifiability: Any claims relating to the benefits/performance of a specific treatment, commercial product, or service will be supported by appropriate, balanced evidence in the manner outlined above in principle 4.
6. Transparency of authorship: The designers of this Web site will seek to provide information in the clearest possible manner and provide contact addresses for visitors who seek further information or support. The Web master will display his/her e-mail address clearly throughout the Web site.
7. Transparency of sponsorship: Support for this Web site will be clearly identified, including the identities of commercial and noncommercial organizations that have contributed funding, services, or material for the site.

8. Honesty in advertising and editorial policy: If advertising is a source of funding, it will be clearly stated. A brief description of the advertising policy adopted by the Web site owners will be displayed on the site. Advertising and other promotional material will be presented to viewers in a manner and context that facilitates differentiation between it and the original material created by the institution operating the site.

The HONcode has been cited as "the oldest, and perhaps the best known quality label" (P Wilson, BMJ 2002;324:598-602). Historically, in other areas, quality standards exist to guide consumers on their choices. The well-known ISO-9001/9002, Good Housekeeping, and the Better Business Bureau are all recognized sources that approve products or industries off-line. In the area of quality rating and accreditation, there is room for more than one group as long as this multiplicity does not confuse Internet users who often cannot distinguish between legitimate and charlatan groups. A team effort among healthcare professionals and governmental agencies can be part of the solution to educate the public about the official accreditation, but a partnership between quality labels is also desirable. An overview of some of these initiatives follows.

In December 2001, the American Commission for Health Care (URAC) began accreditation of health Web sites. Through September 2002, 21 companies received accreditation following a review by URAC based on 50 standards at a fee between $3,000 and $12,000. Twelve Web sites were accredited through December 2002, while the others received, more recently, the 1-year valid accreditation.

Another third-party certification program, the MedCircle project, was first known under the name, "MedCertain." This project's partners are undertaking research to annotate or rate health information and implement the "Health Information, Disclosure, Description and Evaluation Language" (HIDDEL) in XML/RDF to demonstrate and ensure interoperability of rating services. Their results can contribute to the gathering and dissemination of third-party ratings.

Responding to the same concerns about health Web site quality, different medical and professional associations (e.g., American Medical Association), independent nonprofit groups (e.g., Internet Health Care Coalition), as well as governmental agencies (e.g., European Union) have contributed to the preparation of guidelines for health Web sites. While comprehensive, these guidelines are often not exhaustive and are not easily implemented or known by the Web masters of health Web sites. To date, no official review has been performed to assess health Web sites for their respect of these guidelines. However, the Health on the Net Foundation, as an official nongovernmental organization (NGO) with special consultative status to the United Nations with no commercial intent, is in a position to contribute to technical implementation of geographically oriented guidelines. For example, HON could incorporate the European Union Commission's code to its existing list of HONcode accredited European Web sites.

The European Commission code of practice for health Web sites aims for realistic rules and easily digestible criteria for designers creating Web sites, and for end-users building their own opinion on a site's credibility. The core of the code of conduct includes transparency and honesty, authority, privacy and confidentiality, currency, accountability, and accessibility (Watson R. BMJ 2002;324: 567).

With the potential to confuse Internet users, several other accreditation marks, awards, and rating systems exist. Mainly geographically or language-oriented, local initiatives by associations recently emerged, such as the Web Medica Acreditada from the Medical College of Barcelona and the TNO-QMIC in the Netherlands (Bosch X. BMJ 2002; 324:567. Sheldon, T., idem).

Other seals also exist for Web sites on the Internet, mainly to lend credibility to the security of financial transactions or privacy concerns. Two examples are the Trust-e Privacy program (with a specific e-health sublabel) and the Better Business Bureau's BBB OnLine Reliability and Privacy seal.

Based on the rationale of providing a trusted virtual domain of health Web sites, the World Health Organization (WHO) continues to evaluate the "dot-health" domain extension. Divergent opinions have emerged about the actual implementation of this project. It will be interesting to follow its evolution in the near future.

As a conclusion on the multitude of seals, it is important to avoid a monopolistic approach, but efforts should be targeted toward unified actions for the benefit of patients and to avoid confusion. Convergent educational campaigns could help citizens to recognize the accepted "seals of approval."

Search Engines

Most Internet users first approach a subject through general-purpose search engines such as Google, currently one of the most the most popular. These have the advantage of being extremely well known and easy to use. Commercial Web site operators attach much importance to the ranking and placement of their sites in the search results for a given query term, and often resort to unscrupulous techniques to achieve this. In an attempt to thwart abuse and for competitive reasons, search engine operators tend to maintain secrecy about their ranking algorithms. Moreover, media companies like Google do not claim authority in any subject area, and the lack of transparency of their ranking process could, from the scientific standpoint, relegate them to the role of entertainment provider. Public users, however, may perceive search engine results as conferring a degree of legitimacy on the sites listed. And while Google guarantees that its rankings are not influenced by payment from site operators, not all search engines make this claim. In fact, "pay for placement" schemes are on the rise among search engine operators.

Obtaining a page of reliable search results, then, is no easy task. Tools are under development by HON to help information searchers formulate health and medical queries that are likely to yield quality results. This is one of the goals of the WRAPIN (Worldwide online Reliable Advice to Patients and INdividuals) project (see next section). But once the searcher has obtained a results page listing potentially relevant Web sites, what process can quickly unite them with the most helpful information?

"Recent data suggest that the sites most commonly used by patients to find health-related information are the generic portals and search engines (using simple one-word search terms). From the nonphysician perspective, are these then 'best'? It's hard to argue against what the users choose," says David Masuda, Lecturer, Department of Medical Education and Biomedical Informatics, University of Washington School of Medicine.

When people seek information, they don't want to "rummage around" a Web site with the hope that they may find something; they want to go right to it. According to Pew, health information seekers typically start at a search site and visit two to five sites during an average visit of 30 minutes. With search engine results so variable and top placement impossible to guarantee, it is important that quality information be readily identifiable as such.

Medical search engines such as MedHunt and OMNI give acceptable results. HON's most recent survey shows that professionals prefer such specialized search tools (56%), while the greatest number of individuals (44%, with 25% undecided) prefer general-purpose tools.

WRAPIN: The Next Generation of Tools

The HONcode proposes a set of directives to Web publishers with goals of improving the quality of information available on the Internet and helping to identify the Web sites that are updated by qualified people and contain reliable information. However, HONcode accreditation is not sufficient, and our confidence space must be developed. What we must do first is help users where they most need help, that is, at the level of formulating a question, searching for information, and judging the truthfulness of the document found.

WRAPIN, a project of the European Commission, has this goal. This project was initiated and is co-coordinated by HON. The objective of this project is to help in the formulation of more efficient medical questions and to improve current services such as HONselect. WRAPIN will be a federal system of medical information with an editorial policy of intelligently sharing quality, professional information. WRAPIN is defined as a federal system of high-value knowledge in keeping with ExPASy—the proteomics Web server (http://www.expasy.org/). WRAPIN will help in sharing this knowledge, with which the individual can make informed judgments on medical information found on the Web.

The WRAPIN project has two mains axes: the efficient and intelligent search of information and the assertion of trustworthiness content. To assess the trustworthiness of online information, it is compared to scientifically reliable published documents accessible via scattered and invisible databases.

Building on research conducted during the past 7 years by the Division of Medical Informatics (HUG, Geneva) in natural language processing and LERTIM (http://cybertim.timone.univ-mrs.fr/CybErtim/LERTIM/Default.htm) (Marseilles) in semantic representation using the working prototype ARIANE, with HON in information-retrieval technologies using existing tools (MARVIN/MedHunt/HONselect), including new developments with WRAPIN, will offer the user a semiautomatic editorial policy applicable to any health-related Web page or free text.

The WRAPIN system will be able to analyze any medical text or Web page, comparing it with trustworthy scientific articles from visible and invisible scattered databases. The prototype retrieves and attributes the significant MeSH terms (Medical Subject Headings from the National Library of Medicine) found in the entry document, then proposes search keys according to the remote databases to be queried. This phase is the most critical and central phase in the WRAPIN project. Indeed, the quality of the next steps, the interrogation of remote medical databases and analysis of the results, depends on mapping MeSH terms to selected search keys. The prototype already interconnects well-known trustworthy databases such as MEDLINE, MedHunt, HONcode sites, URO database (of the AFU, French Urology Association), and clinical trials. HON's 3400 medical images and videos (HONmedia) representing over 1800 medical subjects, is being integrated. The WRAPIN project is ending in August 2003 and the result will be available on the HON Web site.

Conclusion

The case of online health information begs the question: Is more better? Recognizing consumer demand for choice, we must answer in the affirmative. But much remains to be done to streamline access to the most reliable information and prepare the public to use it.

How can we help the public make use of online resources and minimize the danger of abuse, while preserving freedom of expression and choice? How are we to guide information providers and the public to create an environment of mutual respect and trust?

The Internet favors communication among patient, physician, and pharmacist, and brings disease sufferers out of isolation and into intense interaction. Consensus, based on trust, will arise from the goodwill and efforts of all stakeholders. HON, a neutral body already grouping thousands of online health information providers, can mediate among all stakeholders and, in consultation with governments, the European Union, and the United Nations, is elaborating standards and creating tools to improve access to the best online health and medical information.

The Internet is not an environment conducive to regulation, but one in which voluntary participation, correct behavior, and respect can be rewarded. Tools, adapted to the needs of all types of users, can be made available to increase consumer awareness and create channels for feedback to the professional and governmental sectors. Conflicts of interest can be avoided and consumer awareness increased with improved communication.

We must all learn together to see how we are going to communicate in the future. We are at the advent of a new era in health care and medicine in which users, healthcare providers and practitioners, directors, and managers work together to make efficient use of new information and communication technologies.

References

1. Boyer C, Selby M, Scherrer JR, Appel RD. The Health On the Net Code of Conduct for medical and health Websites. Comput Biol Med 1998;28(5):603–610.
2. Boyer C, Selby M, Appel RD. The Health On the Net Code of Conduct for medical and health web sites. Medinfo 1998;9(pt 2):1163–1166.
3. http://www.hon.ch/HONcode.
4. Pew Internet and American Life Project, Vital decisions, May 2002. http://www.pewinternet.org.
5. Baujard O, Baujard V, Aurel S, Boyer C, Appel RD. A multi-agent softbot to retrieve medical information on Internet. Medinfo 1998;9(pt 1):150–154.
6. Baujard O, Baujard V, Aurel S, Boyer C, Appel RD. MARVIN, multi-agent softbot to retrieve multilingual medical information on the Web. Med Inform (Lond) 1998;23(3):187–191.
7. Boyer C, Baujard O, Baujard V, Aurel S, Selby M, Appel RD. Health On the Net automated database of health and medical information. Int J Med Inform 1997; 47(1–2):27–29.
8. http://www.hon.ch/MedHunt.
9. http://omni.ac.uk/.
10. Boyer C, Baujard V, Griesser V, Scherrer JR. HONselect: a multilingual and intelligent search tool integrating heterogeneous web resources. Int J Med Inform 2001;64(2–3):253–258.
11. Boyer C, Baujard V, Scherrer JR. HONselect: multilingual assistant search engine operated by a concept-based interface system to decentralized heterogeneous sources. Medinfo 2001;10(pt 1):309–313.
12. Boyer C, Baujard V, Griesser V, Scherrer JR. HONselect: a multilingual and intelligent search tool integrating heterogeneous Web resources. Stud Health Technol Inform 2000;77:273–278. (No abstract available.)
13. http://www.hon.ch/HONselect/.

Section III
Telemedicine and Telehealth

III
Introduction: Telemedicine and Telehealth

ROSEMARY NELSON

Telemedicine, the practice of transferring medical data using interactive audio, visual, and data communication systems, is quickly becoming indispensable in modern medicine, healthcare delivery, and education. The telemedicine arena has experienced tremendous growth in the United States over the past few years. The "2001 Report of U.S. Telemedicine Activity," published by the Association of Telehealth Service Providers, which reflects industry trends and promising applications, identified 206 telemedicine programs in 2001, up from 170 in 1999. Responding to the survey were 82 programs operating out of 1278 sites, an average of about 16 per telemedicine network.

On a more regional front, telemedicine is rapidly expanding in the state of Maine, which claims it has become the largest provider of telemedicine services among the 50 states. In a November 21, 2002, issue of the *Bangor Daily News*, Dr. Arvind Patel, medical director of Lubec-based Maine Telemedicine Services, reported that almost 200 sites across the state are using telemedicine technology, and that number is growing at the rate of two to four sites per month. The primary use of telemedicine in the state of Maine has been the transfer of electronic medical data from one location to another, including high-resolution images, sounds, and live video. There is an overall belief that moving information rather than patients is far less expensive than traditional medicine, which requires patients to travel to the provider.

Telemedicine is no longer just a playground for dreamers, technology enthusiasts, and pilot programs. It has become a strategic tool for CEOs, hard-eyed medical directors and administrators, and entrepreneurial practitioners, who raise the following questions: Does it help us address clinical and patient care issues in a more efficient manner? Does it make sense economically? Will it help the bottom line? These questions are still asked, as are questions about reimbursement for telemedicine services and standards. Despite the issues that remain, progress has been made at all levels:

- The 107th Congress (2001-2002) addressed more than 60 different legislative proposals that mentioned telemedicine or telehealth. Several of these legislative proposals received funding in the 2003 funding cycle, such as authorization for the Office for the Advancement of Telehealth (OAT), expansion of the OAT program, and funding to facilitate progress in policy and standards development. It is also encouraging to see that the 108th Congress (2003-2004) has continued this focused attention on deployment of telemedicine to enhance broader access to medical care by all populations.

- In 2002, the Florida Department of Health developed a strategic plan for using telemedicine and telehealth technologies. The plan defines terms and provides guiding principles as the department contemplates using telemedicine or telehealth in the future.

- The American Telemedicine Association's (ATA) attention on the creation of a national telemedicine network for homeland security sparked national discussion among Congress, the Federal Communications Commission, the Department of Defense, the new Department of Homeland Security, and the National Governors' Associations to expand the use of telemedicine in responding to acts of terrorism and natural disasters. The ATA drafted a white paper that served as the basis for the National Emergency Telemedical Communications Act (S.2748), which allowed for states to develop and implement nationwide telehealth networks to enable health professionals to communicate with each other in planning for national preparedness response approaches, and in executing those plans in the event of an emergency.

- The Consumer Awareness Initiative, also sponsored by the ATA, capitalizes on the tactic of "power to the people." This consumer-based initiative promotes the deployment of telemedicine by having consumers voice their desire and demand for telehealth technologies. This tactic is just what the telemedicine industry needs to spark advancement in both the use of telemedicine technology, and to lay fertile ground in establishing billing practices and clinical standards.

The five chapters in this section further illustrate that telemedicine is here to stay, and is becoming a part of everyday life. The section presents a panoramic view of the interactive use of telemedicine and the consumer in addressing disease management and home telehealth; virtual communities; computer-consumer interviewing; and new educational paradigms, such as distance learning for medical, nursing, and online consumer communities. The real-life examples in these chapters demonstrate the positive effects telemedicine technology is having on the delivery of quality patient care, the role the consumer has in the application of the technology, and how ubiquitous the technology is becoming.

8
Models of Health Care and the Consumer Perspective of Telehealth in the Information Age

Loretta Schlachta-Fairchild and Victoria Elfrink

Health care is changing to include an increased emphasis on consumer health services. This shift is linked to the widespread implementation of several information technology advancements. According to the Anderson Consulting Group, the connection between healthcare delivery and information technology forms the foundation of an emerging "healthcare infocosm" (HCI).[1] The HCI is described as the linkage of information technologies, business structures, strategies, processes, and people. The emergence of the HCI has many implications for healthcare delivery including connecting providers, consumers, caregivers, and practitioners with one another and to vital healthcare information at any time, anywhere. While the HCI will continue to develop from today's Internet and related technologies, its proliferation will mark the end of the industrial medicine era and form the foundation of the Information Age of health care.

A Paradigm Shift: Creating Partnerships in Care

Eysenbach[2] described this shift as a paradigm change in healthcare delivery in which the emphasis has changed from the clinical medicine focus of the Industrial Age to the public health emphasis in the Information Age (Fig. 8.1). The information needs posed by the two paradigms are dramatically different. The Industrial Age, often characterized by a high degree of physician control and a low degree of patient power, uses highly prescribed information to help practitioners make decisions for their patients. The Information Age, typified by "consumerist" relationships, draws on practitioner-patient partnerships for managing healthcare delivery by using information that is geared specifically toward each patient.

In a 1999 study, Haugh[3] described the coupling of information technology (IT) and healthcare delivery as a revolution, where the new power of health care is centered with the consumer. The study found that consumers are increasingly using the Internet to seek what they want most: information. This

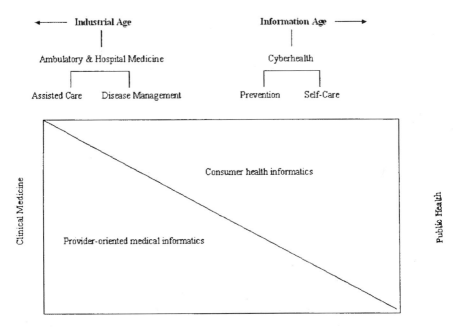

FIGURE 8.1. Healthcare delivery in the Information Age. (Adapted from G. Eysenbach. Reprinted with permission.)

same study also examined the attributes of Information Age health consumers and found that they (1) lead busy lives, (2) have a high level of education, (3) are discontented with traditional healthcare delivery systems including physician care, and (4) believe that new technologies will enable greater access to health care.

While most of the literature to date has focused on the role of the consumer, health partnerships in the Information Age also involve information technology companies and healthcare providers. As expected, information technology companies have embraced the challenges posed by a technology-indisposed healthcare system as they seek new markets. Indeed, over the course of the past 10 years, dozens of private and public Internet companies have begun to transform healthcare practices through the use of information-based services. There are estimates that up to 45% of all Internet searches performed are health care related with the number of adults using the Internet for health information and communication expected to reach 88.5 million by 2005.[4]

Healthcare providers, however, have been slow to embrace the use of information technology in their daily practice. This is a dilemma because studies have found that consumers prefer to access and receive electronic information from their personal healthcare providers than from large healthcare portals. For example, Ferguson[5] noted that most people using the Internet want to use e-mail as method of communicating with their healthcare practitioners. A 1999 Internet user study[6] also supports this trend, finding that consumers who use the Internet would most like to retrieve Internet healthcare information from

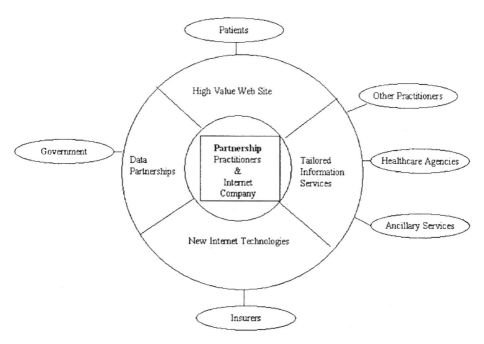

FIGURE 8.2: Proactive Internet strategy. (Source: J. Gruen. Reprinted with permission.)

their personal physicians ahead of national healthcare experts, insurance companies, and healthcare consumer Web sites.

Despite the proliferation of technology tools and the demands of consumers, few healthcare practitioners currently invite e-mail from their patients. The transition among physicians currently providing care in traditional health settings has been especially slow, with studies indicating that less than 5% of doctors who have Internet access in their offices e-mail their patients as part of their practice. Gruen[7] warned healthcare providers of the need to take a proactive partnership role among consumers and Internet technology companies or risk jeopardizing the therapeutic practitioner-patient relationship. He further stated that taking an active partnership role would quickly result in products of value such as enhanced Web sites and tailored information services for patients (Fig. 8.2). Over time, prospective partnerships with companies could also bring about high-bandwidth practitioner-patient communications and management services for the processing of data and control of risk.

Models of Care and Information Technology Growth

While other industries have espoused the use of IT to engage and improve relationships with consumers, health care has lagged behind. It is most interesting to note that models of care and use of IT have developed along reimbursement lines, rather than as independent, business improvement practices aimed at improving the overall healthcare system. The continuum detailed in Figure 8.3 depicts the timeline related to models of care, reimbursement, and technology. As of this writing, consumer-based technologies are just emerging; as yet in the United States there is little to no reimbursement for prevention, remote monitoring, and e-messaging with healthcare providers. However, the surprising yet powerful emergence of forces such as the Leapfrog Group, a coalition of large employers demanding healthcare improvement, may spearhead the thrust toward new models of care based on prevention, remote monitoring, and early intervention. In addition, the nursing shortage and the aging of the U.S. population are also powerful forces that may mandate change in the "acute-based" healthcare system. Currently, Medicare is undergoing a trial of the Care Coordination model, in which capitated payments are made for the entire continuum of care for certain high-cost patients. In an effort to centralize the responsibility for management of disparate costs, a "whole patient" reimbursement model may portend greater involvement of patients in their own treatment and monitoring.

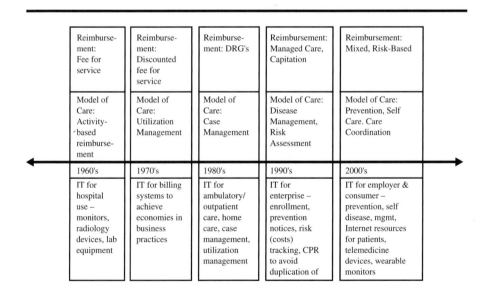

Reimbursement: Fee for service	Reimbursement: Discounted fee for service	Reimbursement: DRG's	Reimbursement: Managed Care, Capitation	Reimbursement: Mixed, Risk-Based
Model of Care: Activity-based reimbursement	Model of Care: Utilization Management	Model of Care: Case Management	Model of Care: Disease Management, Risk Assessment	Model of Care: Prevention, Self Care. Care Coordination
1960's	1970's	1980's	1990's	2000's
IT for hospital use – monitors, radiology devices, lab equipment	IT for billing systems to achieve economies in business practices	IT for ambulatory/ outpatient care, home care, case management, utilization management	IT for enterprise – enrollment, prevention notices, risk (costs) tracking, CPR to avoid duplication of	IT for employer & consumer – prevention, self disease, mgmt, Internet resources for patients, telemedicine devices, wearable monitors

FIGURE 8.3: Models of care, reimbursement, and the growth of information technology in health care.

The Information Age: Realizing Information Technology Products of Value

Even though trends have shown that consumers and healthcare professionals use the Internet for health-related activities, the true potential of the Internet has been slower in health care than in other sectors of American society.[8] Despite the intensive need for timely information, healthcare IT expenditures have lagged behind other industries, and few healthcare organizations including public health offices have integrated the Internet into the provision of care. A 2000 study conducted by the National Library of Medicine found that technical factors, organizational and policy matters, security worries, consumer satisfaction considerations, and concerns over the geographic and socioeconomic digital divide were viewed as barriers to Internet use in healthcare delivery. These barriers notwithstanding, the underlying reason for this limited adoption is a lack of information about products of value. Because the use of the Internet and IT is relatively new in health care and the underlying methods for measuring their benefits are varied and sometimes indirect, it has become difficult to calculate a return on investment (ROI) and in turn identify true products of value.

Consumer Tools in the Information Age

As consumers take a more active role in their healthcare decision making, they are demanding information technology tools that facilitate communications with their clinicians that are interactive and highly personalized.[9] This trend toward accessing highly specific "made to order" electronic information marks a sharp departure from the megaportal Web sites and online services developed in the late 1990s. One term often used to describe this type of personalized messaging tool is the "tailored messaging or information service."

Eakin et al[10] noted that while studies support the importance of information messaging on positive behavior change, there is some confusion about the differentiation among the various terms used to describe a message:

- A *standard* message describes the usual care an individual might receive.
- A *general* message expresses health behavior that is thought of as a "one-size-fits-all" type of intervention.
- A *targeted* message contains healthcare facts that are directed to a specific subgroup of the general population that might have similar specified characteristics and thus similar risk factors.
- A *personalized* message identifies general care for a specific condition. It might have a person's name listed on the information received. The information is general and is not aimed at meeting the individual needs of the consumer.
- *Tailored* information provides essentials that are specifically adapted to one individual's health behavior needs thus creating a healthcare profile.

The authors note that several factors must be in place to create a truly tailored message:

1. Data must be collected from individuals regarding their healthcare characteristics and a health profile created.
2. Healthcare information containing the best-known practices must be available in an electronically retrievable format.
3. A set of decision-making rules created from the information collected from an individual is established to create messages tailored to his or her specific needs.
4. A process must be established for easily delivering the message on the part of the sender and readily receiving the message on the part of the consumer that is clear and understandable to each individual.

Trends indicate that electronic tailored information services will become more mainstream in the Information Age. Because a patient-specific electronic record provides a natural base for individually tailored health messages, online records also open new avenues for health education. On the Internet, it is possible to link personal information to external resources such as glossaries, Web sites, and databases, thus creating true products of value to healthcare consumers.

Telehealth Technology Tools

An increasing number of telemedicine and telehealth technologies are becoming available to consumers. Currently, these tools may be purchased directly by consumers, or may be provided by insurance companies or managed care companies using a disease management approach. Technology tools are also being fielded by home care agencies, in their quest to contain costs under the Medicare Prospective Payment System (PPS). Such technology tools include monitoring devices with or without video capabilities, and with varying levels of complexity and interactivity. Inexpensive independent monitoring devices such as wrist blood pressure cuffs can be purchased by consumers at local pharmacies. More sophisticated devices such as digital peak flow meters not only record readings, but also have the capability to download stored readings to a database for medical/nursing review, trending, and early intervention. Interactive video devices, which run over patients' existing phone lines, are being used to augment or substitute for in-person home care visits and can provide visual assessment capabilities. Integrated home telemedicine systems provide various peripheral devices (such as blood pressure, heart rate, oxygen saturation, glucometer) along with an interactive video capability. Finally, new wearable monitoring devices such as Smartshirt or Lifeshirt, which embed a series of sensors into a common shirt, enable a continuous data stream for monitoring vital signs and physiological parameters.

Information Age Products of Value Already in Use

Given the array of technology tools available, several forward-thinking healthcare institutions have already shifted to the new paradigm for delivery in the Information Age. Healthcare applications are currently being used and evaluated for their ROI. Some applications are focused on addressing a specific health-related need (Table 8.1), while others are multifaceted and offer a variety of stakeholders an integrated approach to care management.

An example of an exemplary multifaceted application is produced by New York City–based Active Health Management (AHM) and is called "Care Engine." AHM's Care Engine is a clinical tool that provides timely analysis of data from physician-patient encounters and identifies patients whose care is not consistent with reputable practice standards. Designed by cardiologist Dr. Lonny Reisman, the technology is aimed at cost-containment based on "clinical excellence" rather than the traditional approach of limiting "resource consumption."[12] Specifically, the Care Engine reviews and analyzes the lab values, pharmacy claims, billing records, and notes. A risk trigger is set in motion if it is determined that there is a breach of care standards such as inconsistent

TABLE 8.1. Information technology-related health care products of value.

Consumer health	Clinical care	Finance and administrative transactions	Public health	Education	Health research
Health Web site	Remote consulation	OASIS and PPS data for home care	Surveillance and detection	Professional education	Databases
E-mail	Medical imaging		Integrating data sources for improved decision making	Continuing education	Linked simulations
Online health records	Clinical transactions				Remote control of experimental apparatus
Patient monitoring and home			Responding to bioterrorist attacks		Publication
			Environmental management		Collaboration
			Prevention activities and targeted treatment		Clinical trials and other research

Adapted from Amatayakul [8] and Chute.[11] (Reprinted with permission.)

diagnoses, missing or incorrect therapies, missing or abnormal lab tests, or dangerous drug interactions. Physicians are immediately notified so that care can be corrected. In 1999, the Care Engine identified 113,633 Empire Blue Cross and Blue Shield members with potential problems such as misdiagnoses or lack of follow-up or preventive treatments.[13] Another function of the AHM Care Engine assists nurse managers in assessing patients, identifying problems, and tracking patient progress problem-by-problem over time and across multiple care delivery sites. Using a set of clinical rules that define standards of care, the system helps the manager to coordinate tasks and other care interventions based on patient specifics and the best-known clinical practices.

Another function of the AHM Care Engine is the Web-based private health record. The AHM engine can update online patient records with timely patient-specific healthcare content including medications, diagnoses, procedures, and care management information. This information can be made available not only to healthcare practitioners, but also to patients. Patients have the opportunity to contribute to their own health care by updating a segment of their record, which includes self-monitoring toward health goals, the use of nonprescription medication, and self-assessment/risk appraisal tools. Integrating data gathered from the myriad of healthcare stakeholders creates a comprehensive yet highly specific patient care portrait that facilitates the use of tailored information management.

Consumer Response to Telehealth Technology Tools

Reports of patients' experience with telehealth and telemedicine technologies are primarily positive. In a report of three case studies of chronic patients in home care, Durtschi[14] reported that patients received more care (i.e., more combined time being visited in person and with telehealth) and they and their families were pleased with the care and attention they received. In an examination of 15 patients receiving home telemedicine-delivered care, Agrell et al[15] reported that although patients accurately perceived major differences between "virtual" and "in-person" home nursing visits, most were still somewhat or very satisfied with the care they received and would recommend home telemedicine-delivered care to others. In a review of 14 pilot or feasibility studies and two studies with 100 or more patients, patient experiences with telemedicine are reported by Whitten and Mair[16]. In general, patients have agreed on the advantages of telemedicine, including reduced waiting times, increased access to care, reduced costs for the healthcare system, the impression that attention is more thorough, and excitement with use of the technology. Reported disadvantages included nervousness over use of new technology, difficulty communicating to providers via the telemedicine interactive system, a tendency to be somewhat less candid speaking with providers via telemedicine, and the experience of emotional distance between the patient and provider.

In general, preliminary studies of patients report positive levels of satisfaction with various telemedicine applications. However, Mair et al[17] report that while patients in general are satisfied with telemedicine, given a choice, both patients and providers prefer face-to-face regular interaction. However, if the choice is between a timely telemedicine visit and an in-person visit in days or weeks, then there are indications that patients may prefer the telemedicine approach. It is clear that the entire arena of satisfaction research, including satisfaction with technology approaches, must be thoughtfully planned and rigorously examined. Asking whether patients are satisfied does not provide significant programmatic information or assess the quality or level of care provided. Use of validated measurements, conduct of appropriately chosen qualitative methods, and detailed study of the topic of satisfaction with technology are all required.

Conclusion

As one considers the Information Age and the ways in which processes, people, and business have the potential to be transformed through information technology, it is important to remember that traditional practitioner roles have to change. Gruen[7] noted that in this era of competition for healthcare dollars, practitioners and organizations must quickly join the Information Age by taking the following steps:

1. Develop an Internet strategy: Practitioners or healthcare organizations need to immediately develop a comprehensive strategy for using Internet technologies to establish their competitive position in the healthcare marketplace.
2. Plan the development of an advanced Web site: Enhanced Web sites should integrate functions and benefits for consumers that differentiate the practitioner or organization from their competitors.
3. Implement a proactive connectivity strategy: Practitioners and healthcare organizations need to manage the data transaction process with other managed care organizations, including pharmacies and laboratories, and digitize these transactions in a structured and logical sequence.
4. Develop a strong data partnership: Care data now stored and capable of being retrieved by information technology tools are extremely valuable. Those organizations and providers that succeed will be those that partner with companies and organizations that can analyze, interpret, and report on this data.

The full implications for how health care will be delivered in the Information Age are years away; however, there is clear evidence that consumers are already increasingly using information technology to manage their health care. Analysts[14] predict that by the year 2006, 65% to 70% of all American households will have appliances with processing power equivalent to a personal computer, thereby facilitating greater access to health care services and education. It seems clear that this paradigm shift in healthcare delivery will continue to grow and that the prolific use of information technology tools will become commonplace.

References

1. Moore G, Rey D, Rollins J. Prescription for the future. Anderson Consulting Group, 1966.
2. Eysenbach G. Consumer health informatics. BMJ 2000. http://bmj.com/cgi/content/full/320/7251/1713.
3. Haugh R. Hospitals and health networks, 1999. Accessed from the New Consumer Deloitte Consulting-In the News. http://www.dc.com/whats_new/in_the news/e-healthconsumer.asp.
4. Cyber Dialogue. Online health information seekers growing twice as fast as online population [press release] May 23, 2000. http://www.cyberdialogue.com/news/releases/2000/05-23-cch-future.html
5. Ferguson T. From doc-providers to coach-consultants: type 1 vs. type 2 provider-patient relationships. http://www.fergusonreport.com/articles/tfr07-01.htm.
6. Cyberdialogue, Inc. Impacts of the Internet on the doctor-patient relationships. http://www.cyberdialogue.com/pdfs/wp/wp-cch-1999-doctors.pdf.
7. Gruen J. The physician and the Internet observer or participant. MD Comput 1999;46–49.
8. Amatayakui M. Is healthcare ready for the Internet? MD Comput 2000;47–48.
9. Kaplan B, Brennen P. Consumer informatics supporting patients as co-producers of quality. J Am Med Informatics Assoc 8(4):309–316.
10. Eakin B, Brady J, Lusk S. Creating a tailored, multi-media, computer-based intervention. Computers, Informatics, Nursing 19(4):152.
11. Chute C. Public health, clinical data, and common cause: information standards as mediating foci. MD Comput 15–16.
12. Active Health Management Fact Sheet. http://www.activehealthmanagement.com/ahmfactsheet.asp.
13. Haughton J. A paradigm shift in health care from disease management to patient-centered systems. MD Comput 2000;34–38.
14. Durtschi A. Three patients' tele-home care experiences. Home Healthcare Nurse 2001;19(1):9–11.
15. Agrell H, Dahlberg S, Jerant A. Patients' perceptions regarding home telecare. Telemed J e-Health 2000;6(4):409–415.
16. Whitten P, Mair F. Telemedicine and patient satisfaction: current status and future directions. Telemed J e-Health 2000;6(4):417–423.
17. Mair FS, Whitten P, May C, Doolittle G. Patients perceptions of a telemedicine specialty clinic and their satisfaction with it. J Telemed Telecare 2000;6:36–40.
18. Robert Wood Johnson, Institute for the Future. Will healthcare join the Information Age? http://www.rwjf.org/iftf/chapter_8/ch8_main.htm

Supporting Literature: Message Tailoring

Bull FC, Krueter MW, Scharff DP. Effects of tailored, personalized and general health messages on physical activity. Special issue: computer-tailored education. Patient Educ Counsel 1999;36:181–192.

Brug J, Steenhuis I, van Assema P, Glanz K, De Vries H. Computer-tailored nutrition education: differences between two interventions. Health Educ Res 1999;14(2):249–256.

Campbell MK, DeVellis BM, Strecher VJ, Ammerman AS, Devellis RF, Sandler RS. Improving dietary behavior: the effectiveness of tailored messages in primary care settings. Am J Public Health 1994;84(5):783–787.

DeVries H, Brug J. Computer-tailored interventions motivating people to adopt health promoting behaviors: introduction to a new approach. Special issue: computer-tailored education. Patient Educ Counsel 1999;36:99–105.

Lusk SL. Test of interventions to prevent workers' hearing loss. Grant 2R01 NR02050-04. Bethesda, MD: National Institutes of Health and the National Institute for Nursing Research, 1996.

Strecher VJ. Computer-tailored smoking cessation materials: a review and discussion. Special issue: computer-tailored education. Patient Educ Counsel 1999;36:107–117.

Strecher VJ, Kreuter M, Den Boer DJ, Kobrin S, Hospers HJ, Skinner CS. The effects of computer-tailored smoking cessation messages in family practice settings. J Fam Pract 1994;39(3):262–270.

Supporting Literature: New Type of Health Care Consumer

Chin T. AMA delegates sort through patient email issues. http://www.ama-assn.org/sci-pubs/amnews/pick_00/tesb0710.htm

Expanding patient-centered care to empower patients and assist providers. Research in Action, No. 5. AHRQ publication No. 02-0024. Rockville, MD: Agency for Healthcare Research and Quality, May 2002. http://www.ahrq.gov/qual/ptcareria.htm.

9
The Convergence of Health Promotion and the Internet

M. Kay Cresci, Roger W. Morrell, and Katharina V. Echt

Many consumers in today's healthcare market take responsibility for promoting and/or maintaining their own health. This paradigm shift from a healthcare provider model of decision making to a partnership model of informed decision making (between the consumer and healthcare provider) is driven by the consumer's access and use of the Internet as an interactive health communication resource. These telehealth information resources are designed to directly benefit health consumers and their families by promoting not only an increased awareness of diagnoses and treatments of diseases, but also the importance of good health practices. This chapter discusses who uses the Internet to seek health information and issues related to its access and use, and provides an overview of several projects that identify and/or address the issues of disparities and health literacy.

Heath Consumers on the Internet

Use of the Internet is expanding at an expeditious pace and this trend will continue. According to a report from the U.S. Department of Commerce in 2002, the number of Americans using the Internet in 2001 reached 54% of the population (143 million people), and it was predicted that more than 2 million users would come online each month following the release of the 2002 report. At that time, it was estimated that more than half of all Americans between the ages of 10 and 55 make use of the Internet. However, the frequency of Internet use falls off steadily after age 55.[1] Although adults in their sixth decade of life and above are less likely to be Internet users, it is important to note that older adults are surfing the Web with growing confidence and destroying myths about their reluctance to use information technology, as will be discussed in detail later in this chapter.

One of the primary reasons that older adults and many younger individuals use the Internet is to find health information. Consumers using the World Wide Web as an interactive health communication resource are identified as e-health consumers,[2] health seekers,[3] or consumer specialists.[4] Findings in the most recent survey (March 2002) conducted by the Pew Internet and American Life Project (PIP) indicate that 73 million Americans use the Web to locate health information as compared to 52 million in the 2000 survey (August). Most consumers go online from home (80%) and are women (72%), ages 50 to 64 (71%), college graduates (69%), with 3 years or more of Internet use (68%). Findings also indicate that half of these consumers seek information not only for themselves but also for family members and friends.[3]

Health consumers access the Internet not only from home but also from work, libraries, and schools. They use the Internet to seek health information because it is convenient; available anytime of the day or night; a global diverse source of information; and can be searched anonymously with privacy and no time constraints. Some of the major barriers to using the Internet include age, education, economics, and concerns about privacy and the validity of the information being presented. Even though the use of computers and the Internet has grown in every income bracket, educational level, age, race, and gender, individuals living in low-income households or those who have little education still trail the national average.[3,5,6]

Fox and Rainie[3,6] found that consumers' use of interactive health communication resources included health Web pages (94%), online health communities (3% to 9%), and online interactions with health professionals (3% to 9%).

Health Web Pages

Health Web pages are visited by 6 million American consumers each day for the purpose of locating information on diseases and treatment, women's health issues, mental health issues, nutrition, fitness, pharmaceuticals, and sensitive health topics, and to access performance reports regarding providers, hospitals, and managed care organizations. Some consumers research symptoms online in an attempt to self-diagnose, but most conduct searches to either supplement advice from a healthcare provider or to understand a diagnosis and its treatment options. Health consumers share the information with their healthcare provider and use it as part of a more empowered decision-making process.[3,6]

Many adults want to learn how to find health information on the Internet. For example, in one survey, middle-aged (40- to 59-year-olds), young-old (60- to 74-year-olds), and old-old adults were asked what they would like to learn how to do on the Internet. All three age groups listed their desire to locate health information as one of their top three choices of the Internet skills they would like to acquire.[7] Data from an additional survey suggests that if older adults are divided into two age groups, that 44% of adults age 60 to 64 and 51% of individuals over the age of 64 who are currently online consumers have accessed health information on the Internet.[8] Of the entire sample, 44% had searched for general health information, 41% searched for information for specific conditions, 21% searched for information on prescriptions, and 13% received health newsletters through e-mail. Other activities included using a health plan site (9%), e-mailing a healthcare professional (8%), using a hospital site (7%), participating in an online support community (7%), using a doctor's site (5%), and getting health insurance quotes (5%). Clearly, Internet users and older surfers in particular are aware of their ability to find medical and a variety of other types of health-related information on the Internet and many of those who have access to the Internet are doing so.

Online Health Communities

The second interactive health communication resource used by consumers is online health communities. Initially developed by health consumers seeking information about the same health or medical issue, these communities are usually centered on a topic (e.g., heart disease, diabetes, asthma, HIV) and include valuable resources from health information and current research on treatment options to self-help and mutual support. Members of these communities exchange information using chat rooms, bulletin boards, or e-mail lists. Members are able to reach out to people not only in this country but also around the world. Common issues and concerns are shared, discussed, and sometimes solved through the practical advice from experienced members. These communities connect people through the convenience of their own home, with no extra cost beyond the cost of the Internet service provider. The low percentage of health consumer participation in these communities is attributed to a concern over protecting one's privacy and the confidentiality of one's personal health data.[9]

Other online health communities available to consumers are health Web sites that provide tools for managing one's health. Many of the sites offer a custom personal health Web site that includes a personal health record as well as a personal health profile created and maintained by the consumer. The site is developed using the person's understanding of his/her health conditions, medications, problems, allergies, and so on. Such a record helps patients concisely explain their health problems when they meet with a healthcare provider. The profile provides the consumer with resources related to their health needs including health Web site and virtual online communities.[10]

E-Mail

The third interactive health communication resource used by consumers is e-mail. Findings from several studies indicate that 3% to 9% of health consumers have communicated online with a health professional.[3,11] This low percentage is consistent with other studies. Health consumers and providers find speed, convenience, utility of managing simple problems, efficiency, improved documentation, and avoidance of telephone tag as positive characteristics of e-mail communication.[12,13] They noted that e-mail is useful to request prescription refills, for nonurgent consultations, and to obtain results from routine tests, provided responses are received in a timely manner.[11,14] In addition, 37% of respondents in the PIP surveys[3,6] indicated that they are willing to pay for this service.

Issues Concerning the Use of the Internet to Locate Health Information

Issues concerning the use of the Internet for seeking health information include searching techniques, trustworthiness of information, privacy, and site design and usability.

Searching Techniques

Findings in the PIP study[3] indicate that most health consumers do not have a specific research plan as recommended by health experts. Rather, they begin a search with a targeted question, then select a search site and take about 30 minutes to follow several links from the search to visit two to five sites.[3,15]

Trustworthiness of Online Health Information

Seventy-two percent of health consumers believe all or most of the health information they find online. They are reassured of the trustworthiness of the information if the advice matches either what is already known or is repeated at several of the visited sites. They do not consider information trustworthy if the site seems to be selling a product or does not clearly identify the source of the information.[3] Little is known about the health consumer's knowledge of groups that provide "seal of approval" for sites that meet standards for privacy, security, credibility, and reliability of health information on the Web such as is offered by Health on the Net Foundation's (HON) code of conduct, Hi-Ethics, and eHealth code.

Privacy

A major concern of health consumers is privacy. African Americans and Internet newcomers show the highest concern regarding privacy.[16] Health consumers fear that others will find out about their activities online.

Health Web Pages

Eighty-nine percent of health consumers are concerned that Internet companies will sell or give away their information, while 85% are worried that insurance companies will use this information to change their coverage. Thus, health consumers want to either maintain anonymity and not share personal information online such as e-mail addresses or give inaccurate online health information.[3,6] Little is known about the health consumer's knowledge related to health Web sites' privacy policies and such groups as Trust*e that provide a third-party oversight "seal" program to alleviate consumers' concerns about online privacy.

Online Health Communities

Privacy and confidentiality is a major issue with online community sites because they require the consumer to provide sensitive information about their health and may collect additional information on the consumer without their knowledge and consent. The information provided to many of these sites is not protected under the Health Insurance Portability and Accountability Act (HIPAA). HIPAA protects information provided only to healthcare providers, health plans, and healthcare clearinghouses,[17] not to such Web sites as eDiet.com, WebMD.com, YourDiagnosis.com, and PersonalMD.com.

E-Mail

The American Medical Informatics Association (AMIA) identified a need for guidelines on the use of e-mail as a communication tool between healthcare providers and their patients within a contractual relationship. Guidelines were developed by a working group of AMIA and address such issues as turn-around time for response, types of appropriate transactions, informed consent, and storage of messages in the patient's chart.[18]

Site Design and Usability

Design and usability of health Web sites is critical to the consumers' ease in finding appropriate information. Yet Web site developers rarely address the characteristics of cultural appropriateness, health literacy, and the age-related sensory (vision and hearing) and cognitive changes of the targeted group when creating their Web sites. This issue cannot be discussed here due to space constraints, but references addressing these issues are identified at the end of the chapter.

The Digital Divide and Health Information

The digital divide reflects individual differences in the ability to access and use information technology based on a variety of factors including age, household income, and education. Seeking health information is equally compelling to older adults of all racial and ethnic groups regardless of income level. The Web's appeal to older adults and various racial and ethnic groups may be determined by the empowerment that results from being an active participant in managing one's health. It has been recommended that to ensure the participation of all Americans in the information revolution, it is important to (1) continue to create access points not only in libraries and community centers but also in nontraditional places such as health centers, assisted living facilities, and low-income senior housing/residential facilities, where people on the cusp of nursing home placement reside and could be kept at higher functional levels; (2) improve educational opportunities for learning how to use the Internet; and (3) encourage the use of the Internet access across locations.

Older Adults' Use of the Internet

Older adults are logging on to the Internet more and more often, destroying the long-held myths that they are afraid and reluctant to use new technologies, especially computers and the Internet.[1,19,20] This should not be surprising, because it has been shown that older adults can readily learn how to use computers and the Internet and retain these skills over time.[7,21-23] Coupled with this increase in use of information technology is the expectation that the number of persons over the age of 60 will increase substantially over the next several decades, reaching 70 million or about 20% of the population by 2030.[24] Because of these projections, it is likely that Web sites developed to entice the attention of older adults will begin to occupy greater real estate on the Internet. Highly visible among these will be Web sites of federal agencies offering social services or health-related information to older individuals, their family members, and their caregivers.

However, despite the popularity of the Internet, retrieving information on it remains a troublesome process. This is the case because most Web sites are inaccessible at some level to older adults even with high-end adaptive technology. For example, very few designers have taken into consideration how age-related declines in vision, cognition, and motor skills might impede accessibility for older adults to their Web sites. It is imperative that these problems be resolved to ensure equal accessibility to social services and health information via the Internet for all citizens. Because older adults utilize health services more than any other age group, it is very likely that they could benefit the most from the Internet as an interactive health communication resource.[25]

Ethnic Groups' Use of the Internet

A 2002 report from the U.S. Department of Commerce found that Asian Americans and Pacific Islanders have higher rates of both computer and Internet use than blacks and Hispanics. Yet the growth in Internet use rates was faster for blacks and Hispanics than Asian Americans and Pacific Islanders, with an annual rate of 33% for blacks and 30% for Hispanics. In addition, black households are now more than twice as likely to have home Internet access than they were 20 months ago. The primary online activities were identified as e-mail (45.2%) and conducting product/service information searches (36.2%).

Little difference has been found among online users from various ethnic groups in relationship to seeking health and medical information.[3,6,16,26] The

U.S. Department of Commerce reported in 2002 that 39.9% of online users connect to the Internet to conduct a health services or practices information search. Findings in the most recent survey (March 2002) conducted by the PIP[3] indicate that there is almost equal interest in seeking health and medical information among white (62%), black (61%), and Hispanic (60%) groups. In addition, ethnic groups have the same concerns related to trust and privacy online. Nonetheless, a digital divide still persists, and one of the primary characteristics of this division is economic in nature, namely computers and Internet access are not affordable, especially in minority and low-income households.

Promoting Health Literacy Through the Internet

Health literacy is defined by the World Health Organization[27] as "the cognitive and social skills which determine the motivation and ability of individuals to gain access to, understand and use the information in ways which promote and maintain good health. Health literacy means more than being able to read pamphlets and successfully make appointments." Low health literacy has been shown to be a major problem that impacts substantially on successful treatment outcomes as well as the financial cost of treatment nationwide. In statistical terms, Davis et al.[28] report that approximately 48% of American adults have difficulty with reading and understanding discharge instructions, medication labels, patient education materials, and consent forms. Sixty-six percent of the individuals falling into these lowest literacy groups are age 65 and older.[29]

Health literacy is an especially significant challenge for patients with chronic conditions such as diabetes, asthma, and hypertension. Findings have demonstrated that patients with chronic conditions have less knowledge of their disease and its treatment and fewer correct self-management skills than literate patients.[30] Thus, it is quite possible that older adults who demonstrate the highest prevalence of chronic disease and greatest need for health care might have the least ability to read and comprehend information needed to function as a patient.

African Americans, Hispanic Americans, American Indians, Alaskan Natives, and Asian/Pacific Islanders have been shown to be more likely than Caucasians to perform in the lowest literacy levels in the National Adult Literacy Survey.[31] With regard to adults age 65 and older, Echt and Schuchard's[32] findings begin to suggest that there is a health literacy gap among older adults and that ethnicity and income in particular may place added disadvantage.

The Internet has been described as having the greatest potential for delivering health information to individuals with low literacy skills because it may have a number of advantages over traditional methods of health information delivery. The nature of the technology allows for health information to be individualized or tailored. The user may selectively combine text, audio, and visual elements to further increase their comprehension of a topic. The Internet can protect the anonymity of the users, thus reducing the fear and shame associated with requesting information from healthcare providers. The Internet can be used at any time, which provides greater access to health information and support on demand. Barriers to direct communication among peers and between patients and health professionals can be reduced through e-mail and chat rooms. Finally, health information can be more widely disseminated and updated immediately.

However, it should be noted that there are negative aspects to the use of the Internet to glean health information that must be overcome to make the Internet a viable source of health information relative to traditional methods. These include (1) inaccurate or inappropriate health information, which could result in delays in treatment or inappropriate treatment[33-36];(2) the loss of trust in regular health care applications[37]; (3) the availability of access to personal data such as health records to other individuals; (4) wasted resources and delayed innovation due to ineffective or inefficient applications; and (5) a widening of the "health gap," because those who do not have access to the Internet will not have access to current information. References addressing a more detailed discussion on the topic of health literacy and the original references from which this section was adapted can be found at the end of the chapter.

Overview of Projects Designed to Address Health Issues on The Internet

Despite the problems just noted with Internet-based health information, there have been a number of successful projects initiated that have utilized online resources.

The www.NIHSeniorHealth.gov Project

One of the more ambitious projects to provide accessible health information to older adults is the www.NIHSeniorHealth.gov project, which began as a joint effort between the National Institute on Aging (NIA) and the National Library of Medicine (NLM) and now includes contributions from a number of institutes throughout the National Institutes of Health (NIH). The project was originally conceived as a series of online short courses based on the AgePage health information brochures that had been developed and distributed by the NIA over the past three decades and were online in text format. It was clear that the health information they contained could be expanded if presented on the Web in hypermedia (i.e., with the addition of graphics, illustrations, photographs, video, and animation). Therefore, the project was reconceptualized as a single Web site containing multiple topics concerning issues on aging with the information presented in various formats.[20,38-42]

In the initial phase of the project, the development team identified a lack of guidelines on how to build easy-to-use Web sites for older adults. Therefore, the team conducted an extensive review of current scientific research and identified three basic conditions for accessibility to online information for the older adult. First, material on Web pages (whether text, graphics, animation, or video) should be viewed or read easily. Second, content on a Web site should be comprehensible. Third, the Web site should be relatively easy to navigate.

A unique aspect of this project was the development of a position paper and checklist in addition to the www.NIHSeniorHealth.gov Web site. The position paper, *Older Adults and Information Technology: A Compendium of Scientific Research and Web Site Accessibility Guidelines*,[20] focuses primarily on three areas: (1) normal age-related changes in vision, (2) normal age-related differences in cognition, and (3) the normal age-related effects on motor skills. All of this information was synthesized into the set of guidelines that was used to construct the www.NIHSeniorHealth.gov Web site. The Web site is now considered a model to follow in order to mediate some of the common age-related declines in vision, cognition, and motor skills that are observed as part of the normal aging process.[43-45] A publication from the National Institute on Aging, titled *Making Your Web Site Senior Friendly: A Checklist*,[46] is also available for Web site developers.

Apostolic Towers: Wellness Center

One of the major challenges in the information age is to make information technology available to all Americans. Morrell et al[7] note that the Web is an important source of social support, communication, education, and services for older adults, and it may be an important link in increasing independent function for older adults. The purpose of this project is to bridge the digital divide by providing the residents of Apostolic Towers with access to computers and the Internet.

Apostolic Towers is a senior high-rise building containing 150 apartments. In 1999, the Johns Hopkins University School of Nursing, Apostolic Towers, and the Southeast Senior Housing Initiative entered into a community partnership to develop the Isaiah Wellness Center, located on the first floor. The purpose of the center is to facilitate healthy aging through providing health promotion activities and social support to seniors. Activities provided by the center include social services assistance, weight loss club, exercise group, brown bag medicine check, diabetes support group, aging gracefully, Bible study group, artists' circle, and a poetry group.

The goal of the computer and Internet project is to develop a model for ensuring that low-income older adults have a chance to share in the benefits of the digital age through a partnership with the Johns Hopkins Urban Health Institute (providing broadband access) and Senior Cyber Net Towson University (providing computer hardware and software). The first phase of the project will explore residents' knowledge of the Internet, interest in using the Internet and for which types of activities, barriers they might encounter, desire for training, and specific training preferences. Using literature on training older adults to use computers, the second phase will involve the development of an educational program to teach interested residents how to access and use the Internet with a focus on e-mail. The artists' circle also plans to review information about local exhibits online and the poetry group would like to use computers for its writing activities. The final phase of the project will involve using the computer training and health literacy literature to develop an educational program to teach interested residents how to search for health information and explore how this new skill empowers them to better manage their existing health conditions and increase their ability to make important healthcare decisions.

An Expert Exercise Prescribing System

In this chapter, we have elucidated the reasons that the use of interactive applications delivered via the Internet can be feasible and advantageous tools in health promotion with older consumers. The possibility of tailoring health information and recommendations results in greater possibility of affecting a change in health behavior. Likewise, using interactive technology for health promotion addresses some of the most common provider-cited barriers for health promotion practice, such as time constraints. Such health information technologies can be delivered in stand-alone format (e.g., kiosks, PCs, etc.) or accessed over the Internet.

Boyette et al[47] developed exercise expert system software that generates individualized exercise prescriptions for older health individuals based on responses given by clients and their practitioners to three different questionnaires. These questionnaires pertain to medical history, functional status, mental status, specific preferences, or determinants that are known to influence initiation of exercise behavior and maximize subsequent adherence. These factors are taken into account by the software in generating a personalized exercise prescription.

A usability evaluation was conducted to determine if older adults are capable of interacting with a computerized exercise promotion interface and willing to do so, and the extent to which they accept custom-tailored computer-generated exercise recommendations.[48,49] The findings demonstrated that participants, once trained with an illustrated manual based on prior materials developed for teaching older adults basic computer skills,[21] were able to complete the computerized items within a reasonable amount of time and with minimal assistance from the provider. Equally important to performance is the degree of acceptability to which older adults, and consumers in general, approach health-promoting technologies. The participants rated the system highly for ease of use and for generating a highly acceptable exercise prescription. Initial work evaluating the efficacy of the software demonstrated that there were greater gains in strength and flexibility (but not in endurance) from pre- to postintervention when compared to the control group who received traditional exercise counseling.

Many stand-alone health promotion applications can be readily translated for use on the Internet. This is advantageous given the leveraging effect that public Internet access can have on the health information divide described in greater detail above. In addition to value-added health promotion for consumers, making such technologies available as a part of daily practice may provide valuable time-savings to health providers. Incorporating evaluation into the development process is an important consideration for developers. The myriad health-promoting software and other informatics available highlight the need to ensure that such tools are user-friendly, accessible, and available for consumers to take charge of in managing their health.

References

1. Adler R. The age wave meets the technology wave: broadband and older Americans. National Press Club Briefing, June 26, 2002, Washington, DC.
2. Cyber Dialogue. E-health consumers are set to transform the health care industry. http://www.cyberdialogue.com/news/releases/1999.html.
3. Fox S, Rainie L. Vital decisions: how Internet users decide what information to trust when they or their loved ones are sick. Pew Internet and American Life Project, 2002. http://www.pewinternet.org/reports/toc.asp?Report=59.
4. Calabretta N. Consumer-driven, patient centered health care in the age of electronic information. J Am Libr Assoc 2002;90:32–37.
5. U.S. Department of Commerce. A nation online: how Americans are expanding their use of the Internet. Economics and Statistics Administration and National Telecommunications and Information Administration, 2002. http://www.ntia.doc.gov/opadhome/digitalnation/.
6. Fox S, Rainie L. The online health care revolution: how the Web helps Americans take better care of themselves. Pew Internet and American Life Project, 2002. http://www.pewinternet.org/reports/toc.asp?Report=26
7. Morrell RW, Mayhorn CB, Bennett J. A survey of World Wide Web use in middle-aged and older adults. Human Factors 2000;42:175–182.
8. Bard M. Cybercitizen health: evolution of the e-Health Consumer. Workshop presented to the National Institutes of Health, March 2002, Bethesda, MD.
9. Toledo SE, Napier M. Virtual health communities: a diabetes case study. SR Consultant Business Intelligence, 2002. http://www.sric-bi.com/BIP/DLSS/DLS2272.shtml.
10. Sittig D, Middleton B. Personalized health care record information on the Web, 1999. http://www.informatics-review.com/thoughts/personal.htm.
11. Sittig D, King S, Hazlehurst BL. A survey of patient e-mail communications: what do patients think? Int J Med Informatics 2001;45:7–80.
12. Moyer CA, Stern DT, Dobias KS, Katz SJ. Bridging the electronic divide: patient and provider perspectives on e-mail communication in primary care. Am J Managed Care 2002;8:427–433.
13. Neill RA, Mainous AG 3rd, Clark JR, Hagen MD. The utility of electronic mail as a medium for patient-physician communication. Arch Fam Med 1994;3:268–271.
14. Couchman G, Forjuoh SN, Rascoe TG. E-mail communication in family practice what do patients expect? J Fam Pract 2001;50:414–418.
15. Fox S. Search engines. Pew Internet and American Life Project, 2002. http://www.pewinternet.org/reports/toc.asp?Report=64

16. Fox S, Rainie L. African Americans and the Internet. Pew Internet and American Life Project, 2000. http://www.pewinternet.org/reports/toc.asp?Report=25

17. Choy A, Hudson Z, Pritts J, Goldman J. 2001. Exposed online: why the new federal health privacy regulation doesn't offer much protection to Internet users. Pew Internet and American Life Project, 2001. http://www.pewinternet.org/reports/toc.asp?Report=49

18. Kane B, Sands D. Guidelines for clinical use of electronic mail with patients. JAMA 1998;5:104–110.

19. Morrell RW. Older adults, health information, and the World Wide Web. Mahwah, NJ: Lawrence Erlbaum Associates, 2002.

20. National Institute on Aging. Older adults and information technology: a compendium of scientific research and Web site accessibility guidelines. Washington, DC: NIA, 2002.

21. Echt KV, Morrell RW, Park DC. Effects of age and training formats on basic computer skill acquisition in older adults. Educ Gerontol 1998;24:3–25.

22. Morrell RW, Park DC, Mayhorn CB, Kelley CL. The effects of age and instructional format on teaching older adults how to use ELDERCOMM: an electronic bulletin board system. Educ Gerontol 2000;26:221–236.

23. Morrell RW. Older adults and the World Wide Web: are we ready for them? Paper presented at the International Conference on Technology and Aging, Toronto, Canada, September 2001.

24. Administration on Aging. Profile of older Americans, 1999. http://www.aoa.gov/aoa/stats/profile/default.htm

25. Marwick C. Cyberinformation for seniors. JAMA 1999;218:1474–1477.

26. Spooner T, Rainie L. Hispanics and the Internet. Pew Internet and American Life Project, 2001. http://www.pewinternet.org/reports/toc.asp?Report=38.

27. World Health Organization. Health literacy. Health Promotion Glossary, 1998. http://www.who.int/hpr/backgroundhp/glossary/glossary.pdf

28. Davis CD, Fredrickson DD, Arnold C, Murphy PW, Herbst M, Bocchini JA. A polio immunization pamphlet with increased appeal and simplified language does not improve comprehension to an acceptable level. Patient Educ Counsel 1998;33:25–27.

29. National Work Group on Literacy and Health. Communicating with patients who have limited literacy skills. J Fam Pract 1998;46:168–175.

30. Ad Hoc Committee on Health Literacy for the Council on Scientific Affairs. Health literacy: report of the council of scientific affairs. JAMA 1999;281:552–557.

31. National Center for Educational Statistics. Literacy of older adults in America, 1996. http://nces.ed.gov/pubs97/97576.pdf

32. Echt KV, Schuchard RA. Characterizing older adults with differing levels of health literacy. The 3rd National Rehabilitation Research and Development Conference: The New Challenges, Washington, DC, February 2002.

33. Goldwein JW, Benjamin I. Internet-based medical information: time to take charge. Ann Intern Med 1995;123:152–153.

34. Food and Drug Administration. FDA warns consumers on dangerous products promoted on the Internet. FDA Talk Paper T97-26, June 17, 1997.

35. Scolnick A. WHO considers regulating ads, sale of medical products on the Internet. JAMA 1997;278:1723–1724.

36. Weisbord SD, Soule JB, Kimmel PL. Poison online: acute renal failure caused by oil of wormwood purchased on the Internet. N Engl J Med 1997;337:825–827.

37. Bero L, Jadad AR. How consumers and policy makers can use systematic reviews for decision-making. Ann Intern Med 1997;127:37–42.

38. Dailey SR. The interactive online AgePage learning project: results from usability testing. Paper presented at the 43rd annual meeting of the Gerontological Society of America, Washington, DC, November 2000.

39. Morrell RW, Dailey SR. The NIHSeniorHealth.gov online learning project. Paper presented at the Second Biennial Conference: Older Adults, Health Information, and the World Wide Web, Bethesda, MD, February 2001.

40. Morrell RW, Dailey SR. The process of applying scientific research findings in the construction of a Web site for older adults. Preconference workshop presented at the annual meeting of the Gerontological Association of America, Chicago, November 2001.

41. Morrell RW, Dailey SR, Rousseau GK. Applying research: the NIHSeniorHealth.gov project. In: Schaie KW, Charness N, eds. The impact of technology on successful aging. New York: Springer, in press.

42. Morrell RW, Mayhorn CB, Bennett J. Older adults online in the Internet century. In: Morrell RW, ed. Older adults, health information, and the World Wide Web. Mahwah, NJ: Lawrence Erlbaum Associates, 2002.

43. Echt KV. Designing web-based health information for older adults: visual considerations and design directives. In: Morrell RW, ed. Older adults, health information, and the World Wide Web. Mahwah, NJ: Lawrence Erlbaum Associates, 2002:61–87.

44. Morrell RW. The application of cognitive theory in aging research. Cogn Technol 1997;2:44–47.

45. Morrell RW, Echt KV. Designing instructions for computer use by older adults. In: Fisk AD, Rogers WA, eds. Handbook of human factors and the older adult. New York: Academic Press, 1997:335–361.

46. National Institute on Aging. Making your Web site senior friendly: a checklist. Washington, DC: NIA, 2002.

47. Boyette LW, Lloyd A, Manuel S, Boyette JE, Echt KV. Development of an exercise expert system for older adults. J Rehabil Res Dev 2001;38(1).

48. Echt KV, Kressig RW. The potential of interactive technology for health promotion with older adults. Proceedings of the International Conference on Technology and Aging, Toronto, 2001.

49. Kressig RW, Echt KV. Exercise prescribing: computer application in older adults. Gerontologist 2002;42(2):273–277.

Additional Web Site Design and Usability Reference

Hanson V, Fairweather PG, Arditi A, et al. Making the Web accessible to seniors. Paper presented at the International Conference on Technology and Aging. Toronto, Canada, September 2002.

Additional Health Literacy References

Echt KV, Morrell RW. Promoting health literacy in older adults: an overview of the promise of interactive technology. Bethesda, MD: National Institute on Aging, 2002.

Eng TR, Gustafson DH. Wired for health and well-being: the emergence of interactive health communication. Washington, DC: Science Panel on Interactive Communication and Health, U.S. Department of Health and Human Services, Office of Disease Prevention and Health Promotion, 1999.

Medicare Right Center. Low health literacy, 2001. http://www.medicarerights.org/perspective01011.html.

10
Patient Empowerment, Cybermedicine, and Citizen Education

PATRICE DEGOULET, MARIUS FIESCHI, MARIE-CHRISTINE JAULENT, AND JOËL MÉNARD

Patient empowerment can be defined as "the increasing ability of patients to actively understand, participate in, and influence their health status."[1] Increased involvement of patients in the healthcare process is one facet of a more global trend of modern societies, where citizens no longer accept being passive about decisions that concern their lives, their environment, or their country. Patient empowerment is expected to improve outcome and be cost effective.[2] At the same time, consumer empowerment is likely associated with the development of technologies that perpetuate or accentuate inequalities between the literate and illiterate.[3] This chapter defends the idea that health information technologies, namely telemedicine and cybermedicine, are necessary but not sufficient conditions of patient empowerment. Change in the patient-physician relationship is a logical consequence of patient empowerment and should lead to cultural changes and significant revision of education and training programs for both health professionals and citizens.

The Scope of Patient Empowerment

Patient empowerment concerns all aspects of medical care. Access to printed and electronic versions of patients' own medical records is a growing but not new demand, both from the patient and physician side. This demand is being increasingly realized as a result of progressive national legislation in several countries.[4-6] For example, a recent act in France (March 2002) allows patients to get a copy of their full medical record without going through a physician.

Patients should participate in the data entry process, but should also be able to request the addition of incomplete information, the correction of errors, and the deletion of private sensitive information (Table 10.1). Information must be presented in an understandable way from the patient perspective. For example, appropriate reformulation of extracts of computerized medical record systems may be necessary to foster patient understanding.

TABLE 10.1. Computer technologies that enable patient empowerment.

Patient empowerment domains	Enabling technologies
Patient record sharing	• Shared data entry and update • Right to access and correct erroneous facts • Right to cancel sensitive information • Adapted report production from computerized patient record systems • Formulation and recording of patient preferences • Automatic trace of accesses and updates of the patient record
Knowledge sharing	• Access to filtered high-quality general knowledge • Diffusion of outcome studies • Shared view of the top healthcare providers • Balanced presentation of investigation and/or treatment alternatives • Focused education (e.g., automatic generation of pertinent educational material from patient individual characteristics)
Shared decision	• Integration of patient preferences in the decision process
Self-care	• Availability of services and sources of information • Randomized studies of self-care versus traditional care • Diffusion of decision support systems to support informed decision and self-care • Acquisition of health products through e-health commerce

Patient information is shared by a growing number of healthcare professionals, including nurses, physicians, dietitians, assistants, and highly specialized technicians. Patients should know who, where, and when these professionals access or modify their records and how personal information is secured.[7,8] Signature techniques are frequently integrated in patient management systems that allow the system to keep track of the different sources of data entry (i.e., write accesses). Following up on all authorized or attempted read accesses raises more complex technical issues. Indeed, read-only access to computerized patient records can be direct (i.e., managed by registering the user identification, the nature of information/function used, and the location of access) or indirect, through the use of statistical query programs. Conflicts of interest between patients' right to privacy need also to be balanced against risks for their environment and eventually the obligation for the healthcare professional to declare certain conditions (e.g., communicable diseases) or inform patients' relatives.

Consumer health information is broadly available through different media and the Internet.[6] Patients desire easy access to valid and understandable medical knowledge.[7] Patients also need to be aware of the availability of resources to provide optimal care (e.g., names of renowned physicians and/or institutions) and the results of outcome studies that compare their efficiency.

Integration of patient preferences into medical decision making has received growing attention from health professionals.[9] Terms such as "informed patient choice" and "informed shared decision making" allude to decisions that are driven by best-evidence. Best-evidence includes not only risks and benefits but also patient-specific characteristics and personal values.[10-12] In the informed model, the patient decides what to do after being informed by the physician of the pros and cons of the different options. In the shared model, the patient and the doctor decide together what action to take. This is in opposition to the more traditional and paternalistic model where the physician alone decides what to do.

Patient preferences apply to the scope of possible structures to be used (e.g., home versus institutional, inpatient versus outpatient, centralized versus distributed care) and the selection of the appropriate investigation procedures and actions (e.g., cost/efficiency, selection of the target outcomes of therapies such as the expectancy or the quality of life). As a precondition to shared decision, patient preferences should be made explicit and the corresponding chapters included in the structure of the patient record.

Access to decision-support tools (e.g., symptom interpretation, individualized risk assessment, prognosis calculation, search for drug indications) can help patients to better grasp their condition, formalize their expectations, and participate in the decision process.[7] This transfer of responsibility from the health professional to the patient has to be balanced with the "broader" objective of medicine—to achieve the highest level of care and results. Patient empowerment does not mean reduced physician liability.

In addition, focusing on a unique model of shared decision making does not represent the adequate answer for everyone. In a randomized trial of personalized computer-based information for cancer patients, 190 of the 715 patients who were asked to join the study (26.6%) refused to participate.[13] Patients maintain the right to not know the details of their case. Patient empowerment also means that some patients may still consider physicians as delegates for their health issues and may concentrate their energy on other aspects of life, leaving their health concerns to the experts. These patients are looking at physicians to make decisions on their behalf, without necessarily sharing with them detailed information that the patients may consider difficult to synthesize and apply to themselves. Different patients might prefer the paternalistic, the informed, or the shared decision model depending on the nature of the decision to be made.[12]

From Telemedicine to Cybermedicine

In a traditional view of health care—for example, through the eyes of physicians or health managers—telemedicine applications were frequently conceived as the computerized arm of the health professionals. Telemedicine applications reduce the risk of misunderstanding between patients and their physicians (e.g., patient information unknown to the doctor, doctor information unknown to the patient, interpretation conflicts) and adverse consequences on outcomes. Computer facilities will be progressively installed into patient homes to facilitate disease follow-up, reduce the costs and risks (e.g., nosocomial infections) of inpatient care, and create an infrastructure for electronic and secure patient-physician communication. Patient participation in data entry (e.g., symptoms[10] and vital signs) facilitates the work of the professionals who are in the best situation to filter the information and make the right decision. Indeed, pioneer applications for the follow-up of chronic conditions (e.g., chronic renal failure, congestive heart failure, diabetes, hypertension, asthma, cancer) or well-defined acute situations (immediate postoperative periods, premature babies) have shown the value of extending hospital networks into patient homes.[14-17]

Cybermedicine, defined as "the science of applying Internet and global networking technologies to medicine and public health,"[18] adds a new dimension to telemedicine. The global coverage of networks extends the scope of information available to patients. In this evolution, physician-physician and patient-physician communications are enhanced by patient-patient relationships (e.g., through e-mail exchanges or formalized discussion groups). Curative and palliative care are complemented by predictive and preventive medicine in which the active patients, not only the healthcare providers, are at the center of the health network. For example, health assessment tools can directly provide the individual with a personalized analysis of his or her lifestyle habits and risk profiles for common diseases, as well as orientations for changing behavior (e.g., stress management, body weight reduction, smoking cessation, etc.).

Self-medication and self-care become part of a global healthcare process in which the gatekeeper role of the general practitioner (primary care) is bypassed by the creation of direct links between patients and specialists (secondary care) from one side, and patients and nonphysicians (e.g., nurses, community pharmacists, patients' groups) from the other side. It also paves the way for a new business, the e-health business, for which providers are looking for future clients in the promising market of citizen-oriented health products (e.g., dietetic and pharmaceutical products, fitness programs, behavioral programs, etc.).

Cybermedicine Is Not Synonymous with Increased Quality of Care

The expected benefit of cybermedicine is increased quality of care as a result of shared decision making between patients and healthcare providers[17]. The reality of this benefit needs to be continually assessed and monitored. For example, the benefits of validated educational information, demonstrated in preliminary controlled studies, need to be systematically assessed, published, and made available through the Internet.[18,19] Indeed, the issue that needs to be avoided is the lack of quality through either excessive or inappropriate information.

Conflicts of interest between the industry that tries to promote high transaction volumes on communication lines or e-health business and the interest of the individual that looks for selected and validated information/health products put a financial pressure on the end users who are encouraged to pay without guarantee of results or a clear refund policy. Unintended manipulation of information—due to lack of professionalism, for example—or intended disinformation diminishes confidence in the health system and may influence patients to make the wrong decisions or to make no decision at all. At the very least, information providers should respect published charts of quality, such as the Health on the Net (HON) or HITI codes, respect conditions of transparency of information sources and exclusion of interest conflicts, and link their materials to published independent evaluation of their quality.

Development of complementary approaches or specific incentives is necessary to reach or involve excluded minorities. In countries in which health care is centrally managed, widespread use of the Internet is likely to aggravate conflicts between patient's expectations and the provision of health care.[20] Quality of care is both the affair of the individual and the population defending the collective interest.

Cultural and Educational Changes

Development of cybermedicine applications represents both a catalyst and a technological consequence of patient empowerment.

Patient Empowerment and Professional Education

To enter into a win-win mode of cooperation with proactive patients, healthcare professionals should be prepared for in-depth revision of their education and training programs and accept deep changes in their attitude with patients. Appropriation of communication and Internet technique is a technical prerequisite for all physicians who need to collaborate with other professionals and patients through health information networks (Table 10.2) Physicians' background on the principle of evidence-based medicine is another prerequisite to be able to respond to the checklists and to the structured questions that might arise from their patients. Knowledge on the general aspects of prediction (e.g., genetic counseling), prevention, and environment-disease relationships should complement highly specialized knowledge on disease prevention and treatment strategies.

Physicians should be ready to direct patients to sources of high-quality health-related Web sites including bibliographic databases, evidence-based knowledge sources such as the Cochrane Library, or dedicated interest groups. Physicians also should share their favorite sources of information with other professionals and patients.[6] Providing information on the Internet is no longer

TABLE 10.2. Patient empowerment and medical education

Medical education	Curriculum topics
Communication technologies	• Aspect of man/machine communication • Local and wide area networks, and applications of the Internet in medicine • Information retrieval (full-text bibliographic databases and knowledge banks)
Computerized medical records	• Patient participation to data entry/update • Patient preference structuring and recording • Security and protection measures
Evidence-based medicine	• Dealing with uncertainty in medicine • Evaluation of the strength of evidence • Critical appraisal and review of the literature • Principle of meta-analyses • Permanent audit of information sources • Development of quality-assured databases and Web sites • Guideline production and management
Cooperative decision support	• Workflow management • Workgroup tools • Multirisk and multidecision support
Evaluation and quality management	• Outcome studies, including alternative medicine • Measurement of patient satisfaction • Cost/benefit analyses

the exclusive remit of healthcare professionals, and physicians should be aware of good materials that are prepared outside of their professional network.[20] Patients cannot express their informed preferences unless they are given information of high quality and pertinent to their problem.[21] Pooled practice guidelines may become an invaluable resource for patients who are likely to accept recommendations certified by recognized medical bodies.

Models of doctor–patient encounters that result in the increased involvement of well-informed patients need to be taught. For example, a patronizing attitude regarding the absolute risk associated with a patient condition (e.g., tobacco consumption, high cholesterol) should be replaced by a more proactive discussion that derives from the calculation of the potential benefit (absolute risk reduction) of drug or nondrug intervention. Physicians should systematically discuss with their patients the pros and cons of treatment options that may have different effects on the patient's quality of life.

During traditional in- or outpatient visits, physicians should find the necessary time to answer the questions of more informed patients and eventually accept and be prepared for more difficult interaction situations and discussions. They also need to accept e-mail correspondence with their patients and eventually do direct patient counseling through the Internet.

Physicians should be aware of the changing expectations of their patients and prepare education materials according to patient interests. Readability of such materials is essential and raises the issue of the development and use of adequate vocabularies.[1,7] Physicians, therefore, should be prepared to devote part of their activity to information production and validation, as well as measurement of patient satisfaction.[22] Through unified presentation models such as the Internet, clear-cut separation lines between traditional and alternative forms of medicine are likely to disappear. Therefore, physicians must actively participate in the scientific evaluation of these alternative health approaches and products that are more and more likely to compete with the traditional practice of medicine.

The new minimum requirement of those individuals who, on the contrary, wish to partly or fully delegate their healthcare choices is to obtain a guarantee that the physicians acting for them have training in evidence-based medicine, practice evaluation, and outcome studies. This kind of physician differs from traditional ones who practice mainly on the basis of their experience, along the line of the authoritarian teaching while completing their initial training. Patients who delegate will not look for assistance in the decision-making process on the Internet; they will look for a list of certified physicians who provide proof of a special way of practicing medicine, based on a continually updated critical assessment of the medical literature.

Patient Empowerment and Citizen Education

Medical education can now be conceived in a much broader educational effort toward the health consumer (Table 10.3). Students in primary and secondary school need to become familiar with communication and information technologies, which, in the long run, will change the perception of future patients, students, and physicians regarding cybermedicine and e-health. Teachers should familiarize children with the broad scope of health-related information available on the Internet and should teach how to discriminate between hypotheses and evidence-based knowledge. Examples of issues that can be discussed include the effect of aging on the epidemiology of chronic diseases, the appearance of new risks (e.g., communicable diseases, environmental and pollution related diseases, the prevention of evitable events, or the promise of new therapies, such as gene therapy).

Equally important is the adequate appreciation by the consumer of the constraints associated with the effective practice of medicine (e.g., costs vs. benefits) and of achievable healthcare objectives.[23] An increased gap between optimal and reasonable care (i.e., taking into account personal or local constraints) or expected and achieved outcomes is likely to be observed in an insufficiently informed population. They constitute a recipe for patient disappointment and litigation.[24] In contrast, adequate and timely information on the hazards of medical practices might both reduce medical errors and prevent appeals against professionals or healthcare institutions. In addition, patient empowerment can foster the acceptance of reasonable care on which the patient and the physician can commonly agree.

TABLE 10.3. Patient empowerment and citizen education.

Patient education	Education domain
Communication and information technologies	• Applications of the Internet in health care • Information browsing and retrieval
General health education and counseling	• Health information broadcasting • Prediction, prevention, counseling, treating from simple examples (cardiovascular risk factors, cancer, genetic diseases) • Medical success stories
Focused education	• Uncertainty in medicine • Quality of information and quality of decisions • Quality of decisions and quality of care • From optimal to reasonable care • Medical error prevention • Security and privacy • Citizen rights and duties
Patient participation and partnership	• Lifelong electronic health records • Models of care (delegation, informed decision, shared decision, self-care) • The pro and cons of cybermedicine and e-health solutions

School is a unique opportunity to discuss the issues behind electronic lifelong health records, patient participation in data entry, access rights, and the principles of data security and patient privacy, as well as current and future national and international regulations.

Conclusion

Cybermedicine should offer both a participating and a delegating model of care, and should integrate the need for equity and health for all through the variety of services it may offer. These different models should be presented and discussed early enough to promote the emergence of a new generation of active and well-informed citizens.

References

1. Bruegel RB. Patient empowerment—a trend that matters. J AHIMA 1998;69(8):30–3; quiz 35–6.
2. Lahdensuo A. Guided self management of asthma—how to do it. BMJ 1999;319:759–760.
3. Anderson JM. Empowering patients: issues and strategies. Soc Sci Med 1996;43(5):697–705.

4. Shenkin BN, Warner DC. Giving the patient his medical record: a proposal to improve the system. N Engl J Med 1973;289:688–692.
5. Schoenfelt S. Next generation: how Internet technology propels the electronic medical record. J AHIMA 1999;70(8):30–36; discussion 38.
6. Shepperd S, Charnock D, Gann B. Helping patients access high quality health information. BMJ 1999;319:764–766.
7. Bouhaddou O, Lambert JG, Miller S. Consumer health informatics. Proc AMIA Symp 1998;612–616.
8. Bruegel R, Andrew W. The CPR: patient empowerment paradigm. Healthcare Inform 1996;13(10):26–28,30,33.
9. Brennan PF, Strombon I. Improving healthcare by understanding patient preferences. JAMIA 1998;5:257–262.
10. Entwistle VA, Sheldon TA, Sowden A, Watt IS. Evidence-informed patient choice. Practical issues of involving patients in decisions about healthcare technologies. Int J Tech Assess Health Care 1998;14:212–225.
11. Towle A, Godolphin W. Framework for teaching and learning informed shared decision making. BMJ 1999;319:766–769.
12. Charles C, Whelan T, Gafni A. What do we mean by partnership in making decisions about treatment? BMJ 1999;319:780–782.
13. Jone R, Pearson J, McGregor S, et al. Randomised trial of personalised based information for cancer patients. BMJ 1999;319:1241–1247.
14. Friedman RH, Stollerman JE, Mahoney DM, Rozenblyum L. The virtual visit: using telecommunications to take care of patients. JAMIA 1997;4(6):413–425.
15. Finkelstein J, Hripcsak G, Cabrera MR. Patients' acceptance of Internet-based home asthma telemonitoring. Proc AMIA Symp 1998;336–340.
16. Gray J, Pompilio-Weitzner G, Jones PC, Wang Q, Coriat M, Safran C. Baby CareLink: development and implementation of a WWW-based system for neonatal home telemedicine. Proc AMIA Symp 1998;351–355.
17. Slack WV. Cybermedicine. How computing empowers doctors and patients for better health care. San Francisco: Jossey-Bass, 1997.
18. Goldsmith DM, Safran C. Using the Web to reduce post operative following ambulatory surgery. Proc AMIA Symp 1999;780–784.
19. Eysenbach G, Ryoung E, Diepgen TL. Shopping around the Internet today and tomorrow: towards the millennium of cybermedicine. BMJ 1999;319:1294.
20. Coeira E. The Internet's challenge to health care provision. BMJ 1996;312:3–4.
21. Coulter A, Entwistle V, Gilbert D. Sharing the decision with the patients: is the information good enough. BMJ 1999;318:318–322.
22. Brennan PF. Patient satisfaction and normative decision theory. JAMIA 1995;2:250–259.
23. Ham C. Health care rationing. BMJ 1994;310:1483–1484.
24. Hurwitz B. Clinical guidelines and the law. BMJ 1995;311:2.

11
Telemedicine in Disease Management

JEFFREY A. SPAEDER

With robust emergency medical services (EMS), tertiary care hospitals, and a plethora of procedure-based specialists, the American healthcare system is well suited to treat acutely ill patients. However, the system is not as well equipped to treat patients with chronic illnesses. This has significant implications, not only for the current healthcare system, since 125 million Americans now suffer from chronic illnesses, but also for the future, as an estimated 157 million Americans are projected to suffer from chronic illnesses by 2020.[1]

The distinctions between acute and chronic illnesses are more profound than the duration of the patient's symptoms. There are also differences in who bears the major responsibility for implementing medical treatment and where that treatment is delivered. Acute illnesses are transient, discrete, and episodic. Treatment is directed by medical personnel, often in a hospital or specialized medical environment, and the patient is usually a passive bystander in the process. Typical acute illnesses include trauma, many infectious bacterial diseases, myocardial infarctions (heart attack), and obstetrical emergencies.

Although, by definition, chronic illnesses last for at least 3 months, in practice they are usually lifelong conditions. The disease may transiently worsen and temporarily transform into an acute illness, but even with effective treatments of these exacerbations, the patient will continue to suffer from the underlying chronic process. Although medical personnel may direct the patient's overall medical treatment, the day-to-day care is delivered not by medical personnel, but by the patient and family members, often in the patient's home. Medications and surgical procedures are important components of treatment; however, patient-controlled components such as diet, exercise, and health-related behaviors are equally important. Although cures are rarely achieved, effective treatment can significantly minimize disability and retard progression of the chronic illness. Typical chronic illnesses include heart failure, diabetes, hypertension, and chronic obstructive pulmonary disease (COPD).

The increasing number of Americans suffering from chronic disease is partially due to the aging population and to improvements in treatment of acute illnesses. Since 60% of all Americans over the age of 65 suffer from two or more chronic conditions, it is not surprising that as the population ages, the number of people with chronic illnesses will also increase. Additionally, advances in medical technology have saved patients from acute illness that heretofore had been fatal, but that have left them with chronic illnesses. For example, in-hospital mortality from acute myocardial infarction (heart attack) in the early 1970s was estimated to be approximately 40%,[2] with many of the survivors being left with some degree of heart failure. However, with the introduction of specialized intensive care units in the 1970s, thrombolytics in the 1980s, acute percutaneous angioplasty in the 1990s, and the use of adjunct medicines, the mortality has been reduced to approximately 5% to 10%, with some clinical trials reporting rates as low as 1% to 2%.[3] As a result of these advances, many more patients are able to survive a myocardial infarction (acute illness), but are left some degree of chronic heart failure (chronic illness). The success witnessed in successfully treating acute illnesses has not been limited to cardiology, and in combination with an aging population, has resulted in a dramatic increase in the number of patients with chronic illnesses.

Because patients battle their chronic illnesses mostly on their own, away from clinicians or medical centers, it is imperative that they become active participants in their care. This includes understanding their illness, knowing and identifying the warning signs of early clinical deteriorations, and initiating treatment when necessary. This level of participation requires patients to be well educated about their illness and treatment. Most patients, however, lack this knowledge and require significant education from healthcare providers. Although it is conceivable that this type of education can be provided during physician office visits or hospitalizations, studies show that inpatient education is not well understood or retained by patients. For example, although hospitalized patients with heart failure report that learning about the anatomy and physiology of their heart failure is the second most important topic to learn during a hospitalization (including the importance of weighing themselves on a daily basis and limiting fluid intake),[4] when they return home, 40% of them are unaware of the importance of performing daily weights and 38% believe that they should drink "lots of fluids."[5] This shows that patients are aware of what type of information they require to care for themselves, but have difficulty retaining the information or correctly applying it. This gap may be due to "information overload" from medical personnel, poor teaching from healthcare providers, lack of follow-up in the outpatient setting, or the inability of patients to contact medical personnel in a timely manner regarding questions or changes in their condition.

Even when patients are well informed about their chronic illness, physiologic changes that predate a clinical deterioration may go unnoticed by the patient. For instance, patients with asthma may have an impaired sensation of shortness of breath,[6] and patients with heart failure may subconsciously adapt their activity level to compensate for worsening exercise tolerance. Both of these physiologic responses effectively mask the worsening symptoms from the patient who is unaware of his own deteriorating health. Therefore, in addition to adequate education, patients with chronic illnesses also require some form of ongoing objective physiologic evaluation to detect early changes consistent with a clinical deterioration, even in the absence of subjective complaints.

Finally, patients with chronic illnesses need frequent contact with appropriate healthcare providers. The ability to receive feedback or longitudinal education from healthcare providers is very important, as many patients either forget what was said during a visit or have new questions after returning home. Unfortunately, it is becoming increasingly difficult for these patients to receive timely feedback because of increasing outpatient delays in scheduling office visits. Recent surveys show that the percentage of patients waiting longer than 7 days to see a physician for an acute medical condition has increased from 22% in 1997 to 28% in 2001.[7] Additionally, there is a disincentive for healthcare providers to spend uncompensated time answering questions outside of clinic when they could bill for seeing patients in their office. The result of these trends is that many patients with chronic illnesses do not have timely contact with or feedback from their healthcare providers.

Patients with chronic illnesses therefore need ongoing education about their illness, frequent objective evaluation of their physiologic condition, and the ability to have prompt, timely interactions with their healthcare providers. To address these unique needs, a new paradigm of care delivery called "disease management" has developed, which has two main components: standardized, evidence-based treatment algorithms and patient-clinician collaborative management of the chronic illness, which consists of the following[8]:

- Collaborative definition of medical problems and goal setting, which requires a continuum of patient education with an emphasis on appropriate diet, exercise, and health behaviors; and
- Close outpatient monitoring of patients and frequent interactions with clinicians including:
  - Ongoing patient education;
  - Efficient ways for patients to communicate with their care providers; and
  - Frequent clinic visits to detect subacute physiologic deteriorations.

Close outpatient follow-up has been the mainstay of most disease management programs. This has been accomplished with frequent visits to clinics staffed with physician extenders such as nurse case managers, nurse practitioners, or physician assistants who are supervised by a physician. During these visits, patients are evaluated for any evidence of clinical deterioration, educated about their illness, and given feedback about their health behaviors. Studies have shown that these approaches are very effective, most notably in heart failure where rehospitalization rates, mortality, and overall medical costs have been shown decreased with disease management interventions.[9]

Despite the success of these disease management programs, it has been difficult to expand them to the increasing number of patients who would benefit from them. One of the problems is that these programs require significant face-to-face interactions between patients and healthcare providers. This requires patients to regularly travel to the clinic, which imposes a significant burden especially for those who are frail or live in geographically remote areas. Another is that disease management programs are labor intensive and require staffing with high-cost personnel who are in increasingly short supply, especially in some regional areas. For these reasons, interest has developed about utilizing telemedicine as an adjunct to expand the reach of disease management programs by connecting the patient from their home to the clinician's office. This would not only reduce the patient's travel burden, but also allow clinicians to administer care to areas that might otherwise lack the required expertise. This theory is bolstered by studies showing that telephone outreach can substitute for some clinic visits.[10]

Synchronous and Asynchronous Telemedicine Systems

Although a variety of telecommunication media can be employed for telemedicine systems, in general these systems link clinicians and patients together synchronously or asynchronously. Systems that provide a synchronous or "serial" link allow one clinician to interact with one patient at a time. This often necessitates a predetermined appointment for the interaction to occur so that both parties are available. Although this approach lessens patients' travel burden, it is still labor-intensive. In general, "serial" systems are video-based, either with direct video links or streaming video through the Internet.

Telemedicine systems that operate asynchronously or "in parallel" allow one clinician to monitor multiple patients simultaneously. These systems are partially or fully automated and usually have a computer system interacting with the patients. Using predetermined algorithms, these automated systems supplant the routine monitoring of patients and notify appropriate personnel when problems are detected. Although the degree of personal clinician interaction varies with these systems, by necessity it is limited compared to face-to-face interactions. Personnel costs are decreased with these systems, and patient monitoring, albeit automated, can be increased. These systems often employ store-and-forward technology.

Video-Based Systems in Disease Management

Most video-based systems link clinicians to patients using a two-way interactive video system. Compatible video and display equipment must be deployed in both the patient's home and the clinician's site. Video interactions must be prescheduled so that both the patient and clinician are prepared to simultaneously interact with the system. The interactions between clinicians and patients are reminiscent of typical office-based visits with the clinician obtaining an interval history and providing real-time feedback and education. There are three general types of these video-based systems:

1. Videophones: These commercially available pieces of equipment can be used by patients and clinicians to interact with each other. The videophone is basically a telephone bundled with a modem and video camera. It is easy to use, and simple to plug into an existing telephone outlet. Because most commercially available videophones use standard video compression technology (H.324), the patient and healthcare provider do not need to use the same brand of device. Despite the ease of installation and use, videophones have not been embraced by disease management telemedicine programs because many patients find that the screens are too small, lack definition, or have screen-refresh speeds that are too slow. Although the cost of videophones is decreasing, at approximately $400 per device, they are often too expensive for the disease management environment.

2. Customized video conferencing systems: Several groups have attempted to overcome the deficiencies of videophones by combining off-the-shelf video equipment, which is easier for patients to use, into a single system. These systems use higher-definition video cameras, larger monitors (typically 15 inch or greater), CODEC, modem, and video compression software. These features dramatically increase patient usability compared with videophones; however, they occupy significantly more space in the patient's home. The increased size of the equipment also decreases the mobility of these systems. Most of these "improved" systems have been constructed by researchers at academic research centers and are not commercially available. Nevertheless, they offer insights into the necessary components of a more patient-friendly video-based system. However, because these systems are locally developed and cannot take advantage of economies of scale for production, they tend to be more expensive than videophones.

3. Commercially available integrated video systems: These systems combine the "plug and use" simplicity of the videophone with some of the features of the customized systems. A monitor intermediate in size between a videophone and standard television monitor is integrated into a single device with a video camera, CODEC, modem, and peripheral medical equipment such as a blood pressure cuff and stethoscope. At the healthcare provider's office, a similar device is required that allows the clinician to see and hear the patient and take readings from the peripheral medical devices. Physiologic data such as readings from the blood pressure cuff or the audio component of the stethoscope are transmitted separately from the audio and video data.

With these systems, clinicians can nearly replicate a complete physical examination. Like the other video-based systems, these integrated systems require that the clinician and patient schedule the video interaction in advance so that they can be simultaneously connected.

All three of these video-based systems are highly effective for patient education and monitoring patient activity, especially when this activity involves using medical devices or performing medical tasks such as changing wound dressings, correctly using a blood pressure cuff, or connecting intravenous pumps to indwelling catheters. The addition of peripheral medical equipment may also be very beneficial in specific circumstances; with the exception of a stethoscope, most readings can be transmitted by video and do not require a separate data channel.

Patient acceptance of these systems has been varied. Many patients feel comfortable with these "virtual visits" since the interaction is similar to a routine doctor's office visit. However, the technology can be intimidating to some patients, and the image quality can be a significant issue as transmission of images over low-bandwidth plain old telephone system (POTS) lines can be problematic. Although some groups report that screen-refresh rates of two frames per second are acceptable to patients, rates of at least eight screens per second are more reasonable. In rural communities where POTS lines may provide lower bandwidth, it may be difficult to achieve these rates, and as a result image quality may be distracting for patients.

Although adequate video quality can be difficult to achieve, it can bring other unanticipated concerns since some patients sometimes find it intrusive. For instance, despite the fact that these systems require simultaneous patient- and clinician-initiated connections, some patients have concerns that the video system could be secretly activated, allowing the clinician to view the patient's home. In several instances, decidedly low-tech approaches were required to overcome these fears, including placing a towel over the patient's video camera when it was not in use.

Finally, the larger the size of the telecommunications equipment, especially the video screen, the easier it is for patients to use these systems. On the other hand, the larger the screen, the more space it occupies in the patient's home, and the less mobile it may be. For this reason, patients' use of these video systems may be limited to their homes. This can be a significant drawback since many patients with chronic conditions are anxious about traveling for fear that their health may worsen without familiar medical personnel nearby for assistance. Although telemedicine can potentially overcome this problem, if the system cannot be easily transported, it is of limited value.

One of the major difficulties with disease management programs is their difficulty in treating large numbers of patients. Because all of the described video-based systems still require a one-to-one interaction between a single patient and a single clinician, they are not well suited to provide care to large numbers of patients. To address this issue, telemedicine systems would need to become partially automated so that the system could interact with multiple patients simultaneously. Since by definition there cannot be a real-time interaction between a patient and a clinician in an automated system, there is no need for synchronous telecommunication. Rather "store-and-forward" systems can be employed.

Store-and-Forward Systems in Disease Management

Store-and-forward devices ask the patient a series of questions, record (store) the answers, and then transmit (forward) the data to a centralized, and often computerized, collection center. In the case of computerized collection centers, automated algorithms are often utilized to evaluate the data and notify healthcare providers of any irregularities. These systems allow healthcare providers to passively monitor large numbers of patients and efficiently identify patients whose health is deteriorating.

Most store-and-forward systems have a communication device located in the patient's home that is usually connected to the patient's telephone outlet. On a daily or other predefined basis, a centralized computer server downloads a series of questions to the device. These questions are then submitted to the patient to answer. The communication device either displays the questions on a LCD screen or voice files are played. These devices often have buttons with which patients respond to the questions. Once the patient has answered the questions, the device stores the answers and either immediately transmits the data or transmits it at a later time to a central server. The data are then stored in a database in a highly structured format that can be queried and reviewed by a clinician.

Some of these in-house store devices also have peripheral medical equipment incorporated into the device such as scales, automated blood pressure cuffs, and glucometers. These devices store any patient measurements and then transmit these values with the patient's other responses, allowing the healthcare provider to correlate patient symptoms with physiologic parameters. The questions asked by these devices are either hard-wired into the home device at the time of installation or downloaded from the central server each time the device connects to the server. The device-server connection therefore is a two-way, asynchronous interaction.

One of the problems with any telemedicine system that requires patient interaction with a device is that patients must be in close proximity to the device, or they must carry it with them when traveling. Additionally, some patients are reluctant to have specialized telemedicine devices in the house because of concern about the "stigma" of appearing ill. Finally, systems that rely on an in-home device can be expensive and are more likely to break than a system that does not require the use of a telemedicine device.

Because patients primarily interact with a computer in store-and-forward systems, there has been concern that patients would dislike interacting with a computer. Although some patients find the devices impersonal, most like the ability to interact with the system at their convenience. Furthermore, many patients more readily admit lapses in their behavior to a computer than to a clinician and therefore a computer interaction may be more fruitful than a one-on-one interaction. Finally, even when patients sense that the interaction is impersonal, if it is incorporated into the disease management program as an additional way to interact with clinicians, rather than as a substitute for personalized care, they are often receptive to using it and see it as an added benefit. If, however, the system is not properly integrated into the disease management program and clinicians are not responsive to changes in the patients' health, consumers will view the system as a frustrating obstacle and will not use it.

Unlike video-based telemedicine systems, patients are able to interact with store-and-forward systems at their convenience. Travel is also easier with a store-and-forward device because much less equipment is needed than with a video-based system. Experience shows that patients with chronic illnesses are reluctant to travel away from home because of the fear of suffering a deterioration in their health. However, when given easily transported devices, they are more likely to travel. Systems like TeleWatch, which requires no telemedicine device, are the easiest to use by traveling patients.

Internet-Based Systems

The Internet is increasingly being evaluated to provide telemedicine in disease management programs. This is a natural outgrowth of the fact that consumers who use the Internet are increasingly using it to obtain health information. A recent Harris Poll revealed that 80% of all people online use the Internet to look for health information.[11] Patients are also interested in incorporating the Internet into the delivery of their medical care. Sixty-six percent of patients report an interest in a "virtual visit" for simple medical problems, and many patients have a "strong" interest in communication with their physician via e-mail.[12] This has prompted at least one managed care organization to reimburse physicians who respond to patient e-mails.[13]

The Internet can provide a medium for both synchronous video-conferencing using digital video cameras as well as store-and-forward devices. In this respect, Internet-based telemedicine is very similar to the previously mentioned video-based and store-and-forward systems. However, unlike the other telemedicine media, the Internet also provides an additional method of communication using e-mail. The Internet also offers access to the World Wide Web and the educational resources that it provides. Therefore, the strength of Internet-based telemedicine systems is that it offers a platform that can include both video-based and store-and-forward systems, as well as additional educational and communication resources.

Because of the educational resources available on the Internet, there has been interest in using it to make patients more self-reliant in managing their illness. The IDEATel Project is the most ambitious of these attempts.[14] In this project, rural patients with diabetes in New York State are provided with Internet access and customized computers that have digital cameras and integrated durable medical equipment. Blood glucose readings are stored and then relayed to a central facility by the system. Previously scheduled video-interactions can also be performed using Internet video-conferences with screen rates of eight per second over POTS lines. Patients can also interact with healthcare providers via e-mail and access medical information over the Internet. The goal is to monitor patients using store-and-forward technology, educate patients about their illness, evaluate any clinical problems using the video-conferencing capability, and transition patients into increasing self-reliance with Web-based educational materials instead of reliance on video interactions.

IDEATel highlights the potential synergy of a Web-based telemedicine system. It also has shown some of the potential difficulties with the Internet. First, as of 2001, only 44% of Americans had home Internet access, and only approximately 15% of people over the age of 65 have Internet access at home.[15] Although the number of elderly consumers with Internet access is expected to increase in the future, the lack of uniform Internet access makes near-term deployment of Internet-based telemedicine problematic. Even for patients with Internet access, the incorporation of video cameras and peripheral medical equipment can be an obstacle. For this reason, the IDEATel program provides a "locked" computer system that does not allow reconfiguration by the patient, which prevents accidental tampering or disabling of the system. It is likely that future Internet-based systems will require similar precautions to prevent the computer from being compromised by viruses or inappropriate tampering with the system.

Consumer Satisfaction

Before patients can critically evaluate a telemedicine system, they must first use the system. Their willingness to use a telemedicine system is influenced by their motivation at the time they are approached about using a telemedicine device. In general, patients who have had a recent decline in their health such as a new diagnosis of an illness or a recent hospitalization are significantly more willing to use a telemedicine system than patients whose health is stable. Additionally, patients who are approached in person by a healthcare provider are significantly more likely to use a telemedicine system. Therefore, although the goal of telemedicine is to interact with patients at a distance, healthcare providers must do at least part of the initial interaction with patients in person. The initial contact may be with the patient's physician during a clinic visit, or with other healthcare providers who interact with a patient who has been hospitalized or who has received a new diagnosis. A telemedicine system that relies on anonymous healthcare providers contacting a patient with unsolicited telephone calls or mailings is unlikely to sufficiently motivate patients to use a telemedicine system. This is particularly true of elderly patients who are very reluctant to share any medical information in the absence of an established medical relationship because of concerns of fraud.

Once patients agree to participate in a telemedicine disease management program, they routinely report a high level of patient satisfaction with the program.[16,17] When asked, patients often respond that these systems are "useful,"[18] and in some circumstances that the telemedicine interaction made them feel "as good as a clinic visit" and that it could be used "to avoid clinic visits."[10] They also report more specific comments that generally fall into three categories[16]:

- Increased sense of security: a feeling that they were receiving more time and attention from healthcare providers;
- Ease of interacting with healthcare providers: reduction of travel time and hassles of commuting; and
- Better understanding of their illness.

Despite these anecdotal reports, rigorous statistical analysis of patient satisfaction has been hampered by the relatively small size of most studies and lack of standardized satisfaction metrics. Authors attempting to perform meta-analysis of the existing data have therefore been unable to draw general inferences and are hesitant to report any conclusions regarding patient satisfaction.[18] Interesting, however, is the observation that patients more fully appreciate the benefits of using a telemedicine system once they have used it.[10]

Satisfaction with video-based systems is highly dependent on the quality of the video, and poor image quality can significantly impact the patient's perception of the system. Image quality includes the screen-refresh rate and picture delay. Although there are reports that screen-refresh rates as low as two per second have been used successfully, most patients will find refresh rates lower than 10 per second to be unacceptable.[19] A picture delay of 0.8 seconds is acceptable, but delays of less than 0.4 seconds are preferred by patients.

Effectiveness of Telemedicine Systems

A variety of telemedicine systems have been used in disease management programs. Which of these systems will predominate in the future is unclear. The fact that Internet-based systems can combine store-and-forward and/or video capabilities with e-mail and educational resources may ultimately make it the platform of choice for disease management. However, because the vast majority of Americans with chronic illnesses do not have home Internet access, it is unlikely that the Internet will become the dominant form of telemedicine in the near future. Therefore, the prime area of current competition in the disease management field is between store-and-forward systems and video-based systems.

Although definitive studies comparing video-based versus store-and-forward systems do not yet exist, several small studies offer interesting findings. The first was a year-long study involving 20 English patients with heart failure randomized to either standard care (10 patients) or disease management (10 patients) using a telemedicine system that combined a video-over-POTS combined with a store-and-forward device that monitored pulse, blood pressure, and weight.[20] Patients were requested to take their pulse, blood pressure, and weight daily, which were transmitted by the store-and-forward device. Additionally, they had regularly scheduled videoconferences with a healthcare provider. During the course of the study, patients recorded their weight 75% of the time and their blood pressure 90% of the time. Initially, they had comparable adherence rates with prescheduled videoconferences. However, after 6 months, the rates of videoconferencing dropped precipitously despite ongoing adherence with the store-and-forward modality.

Another small study involved 37 patients with heart failure.[21] Subjects were randomized between usual care (12 patients), frequent telephone calls from a healthcare provider (12 patients), or outpatient monitoring using a video-based system with integrated medical equipment (13 patients). Patients were followed for 6 months, after which there was a dramatic decrease in hospital admissions and overall medical charges between the control group and the other two interventions. However, although there was a trend toward decreased medical expenses with the video-based system compared with the telephone-only group, this difference was not statistically significant. Therefore, there was little additional benefit derived from the videoconferencing capability compared to the telephone group.

These studies suggest that in long-term disease management situations, it may be difficult for patients to maintain frequent video-based interactions with healthcare providers. Furthermore, it is debatable how much the video component adds in a disease management setting. Given the added expense of video-based systems, it is unlikely that they can justify the additional costs compared with store-and-forward systems. It is also significantly more expensive to staff systems that rely on video systems than store-and-forward devices. Therefore, it is likely that future disease management programs will turn to store-and-forward devices as the primary telemedicine device. However, for certain groups of patients who require intensive monitoring or education, video-based systems may be preferable.

How Telemedicine Fits into the Healthcare Delivery System

The early history of telemedicine has been technology-driven. Great effort has been taken to maximize data transmission, but significantly less effort has gone into effectively incorporating these devices into a healthcare delivery system. Unfortunately, it is the effective integration of the telemedicine system into the routine care of patients that is more important than the particular technology used in the telemedicine device. In particular this integration requires:

1. Correctly identifying appropriate patients who would benefit from telemedicine. This is a question not only of compliance and technical aptitude, but also of prognosis and potential for future clinical decomposition and cost savings.

2. Incentivizing patients to continue using the telemedicine system. Patient motivation is very important to the continued success of a telemedicine program. Although patients may be motivated when they are ill, it is often challenging to encourage their use when they are feeling well.

3. Enabling healthcare providers who staff the telemedicine system to make treatment changes. Since these systems are often directly monitored by nurses or physician assistants, it is important that they have either the direct ability to make appropriate medical interventions for patients or an unimpeded process by which they can have physicians make the necessary changes. It does little good for a clinician to detect a change in a patient's medical condition without the ability to make appropriate interventions.

Limitations to Deployment of Telemedicine Systems for Disease Management

Healthcare entities will employ telemedicine systems in disease management if it is economically rational. Entities at full financial risk for their patients will invest in telemedicine only when irrefutable research evidence points to its financial and clinical advantages. Unfortunately, this level of conclusiveness does not yet exist in the literature, although there are strong indications that such a conclusion is inevitable.

For entities not at financial risk for patient expenses, insurance or government reimbursement will be required before healthcare providers begin using telemedicine systems. Without such reimbursement, it is not economically rational for these entities to provide telemedicine disease management, especially since these programs might result in reduced healthcare utilization, which would ultimately result in reduced revenues for the entity.

Conclusion

As evidence accumulates that telemedicine in combination with disease management reduces morbidity and medical cost, telemedicine will become a routine component of outpatient management. Because they are cost-effective and leverage the time of a relatively small number of clinicians to monitor the health of large numbers of patients, it is likely that store-and-forward devices will be used for a large percentage of patients. Video-based systems will likely be used for selected patients who are either medically complex or particularly geographically isolated. The Internet will likely be the medium of choice in the distant future, although store-and-forward devices in the near term will need to employ POTS lines. Store-and-forward devices that have integrated durable medical equipment will have some advantages with ease of patient use; however, telephone-only systems will have significantly lower costs, increased mobility, and ease of large-scale deployment.

The three areas of development that will have the greatest impact upon patients will be:

1. Effective patient interfaces that ease patient data entry while monitoring appropriate medical data;
2. Methods of maximizing patient adherence including outgoing patient messaging and financial incentives; and
3. Patient education incorporated into the telemedicine system. A certain component will likely be automated so that patients could learn how better to care for themselves (i.e., increase their "self-efficacy"). This may include reinforcing healthy behaviors, diet, exercise, ability to detect changes in their medical condition, and even how to make appropriate near-term changes in their treatment to account for changes in their condition.

With these areas of development in addition to a robust telemedicine system, patients will be better informed about their illness and have increased access to their healthcare providers, and clinicians will be better able to monitor patients for early clinical deteriorations and minimize the side effects of interventions regardless of the location of the patient. This should increase the patient's quality of life, while reducing medical expenses.

References

1. Partnership for Solutions. Better lives for people with chronic conditions. Baltimore, MD: 2002.
2. Pohjola-Sintonen S, Siltanen P, Haapakoski J, Romo M. The mortality and case fatality rates in acute myocardial infarction in Finland. The results of Helsinki Coronary Register during 1970-1977. Eur Heart J 1987;8(4):354–359.
3. Antoniucci D, Valenti R, Migliorini A, et al. Abciximab therapy improves 1-month survival rate in unselected patients with acute myocardial infarction undergoing routine infarct artery stent implantation. Am Heart J 2002;144(2):315–22.
4. Hagenhoff B, Feutz C, Conn V, Sagehorn K, Mornanville-Hunziker M. Patient education needs as reported by congestive heart failure patients and their nurses. J Adv Nurs 1994;19:685–690.
5. Ni H, Nauman D, Burgess D, Wise K, Crispell K, Hershberger R. Factors influencing knowledge of and adherence to self-care among patients with heart failure. Arch Intern Med 1999;159:1613–1619.
6. Veen JC, Smits HH, Ravensberg AJ, Hiemstra PS, Sterk PJ, Bel EH. Impaired perception of dyspnea in patients with severe asthma. Relation to sputum eosinophils. Am J Respir Crit Care Med 1998;158(4):1134–1141.
7. Strunk B, Cunningham P. Treading water: Americans' access to needed medical care, 1997-2001. Center for studying health system change, Washington, DC, March 2001.
8. Von Korff M, Gruman J, Schaefer J, Curry S, Wagner E. Collaborative management of chronic illness. Ann Intern Med 1997;127:1097–1102.

9. Rich M. Heart failure disease management: a critical review. J Cardiac Failure 1999;5(1):64–75.
10. Wasson J, Caudette C, Whaley F, Sauvigne A, Baribeau P, Welch H. Telephone care as a substitute for routine clinic follow-up. JAMA 1992;267:1788–1793.
11. Taylor T. Cyberchondriacs update. Harris Poll #21, May 1, 2002.
12. Grover F, Wu D, Blanford C, Holcomb S, Tidler D. Computer-using patients want Internet services from family physicians. J Fam Pract 2002;51(6):570–572.
13. Smith S. Internet visits: a new approach to chronic disease management. J Med Pract Manag 2002;17(6):330–332.
14. Starren J, Hripcsak G, Sengupta S, et al. Columbia University's informatics for diabetes education and telemedicine (IDEATel) project. J Am Med Infrom Assoc. 2002;9:25–36.
15. Department of Commerce. A nation online. Washington, DC: Department of Commerce, 2002.
16. Dimmick S, Mustaleski C, Burgiss S, Welsh T. A case study of benefits ant potential savings in rural telehealth. Home Healthcare Nurse 2000;18(2):125–135.
17. Shah N, Der E, Ruggerio C, Heidenreich P, Massie B. Prevention of hospitalizations for heart failure with an interactive home monitoring program. Am Heart J 1998;135:373–378.
18. Mair F, Whitten P. Information in practice. BMJ 2000;320:1517–1520.
19. Fulmer T, Feldman P, Kim T, et al. An intervention study to enhance medication compliance in community-dwelling elderly individuals. J Gerontol Nurs 1999;25(8):6–14.
20. Lusignan S, Wells S, Johnson P, Meredith K, Leatham E. Compliance and effectiveness of 1 year's home monitoring: the report of a pilot study of patients with chronic heart failure. Eur J Heart Failure 2001;3:723–730.
21. Jerant A, Azari R, Nesbitt T. Reducing the cost of frequent hospital admissions for congestive heart failure. Med Care 2001;39:1234–1245.

12
The Medical Traveler Abroad: Implications for Telemedicine

RONALD C. MERRELL

In preparation for yet another long research trip to the jungle, I pack my lisinopril, 81-mg aspirin tablets, Zantac, allergy medicines, and ibuprofen, and consider taking my blood pressure cuff to monitor my medication. I am not a hypochondriac. I am just a 50-plus-year-old American and taking less than the average medication number of nine for my age.[1] I have a wonderful primary-care physician and access to a comprehensive medical system in which I have great confidence and long experience. My comfort with health care in the United States is not simply because I am a physician, but because of my experiences as a patient. Outside the United States, I could report my medical history to another physician with fair accuracy and might even manage in a few languages other than English. Over many years I have learned a lot about the U.S. health system that might be taken for granted by most Americans, and I have a fair knowledge of the many systems in place in other countries.

Last night a friend called to discuss a trip to England. She has metastatic colon cancer, and at age 80 she believes this may be an important trip to a destination that has brought her much joy over a long life. She wanted advice about how to manage her chemotherapy and other medical issues while traveling. She has a superb medical and surgical team, but is somewhat perplexed about some of the special issues of travel as a patient. Last summer my niece, a newly diagnosed diabetic, went to Europe with classmates and graduated from the close supervision of her parents to self-sufficiency in monitoring her glucose and administering insulin. She also was equipped with instructions on resources for health care while abroad.

We often see people in the airport preparing for foreign travel who seem far removed from the robust young people featured in travel ads. They are in wheelchairs, supported by oxygen, and many require considerable physical assistance. Yet they are traveling long distances and may be entering a truly alien landscape of medical response, relative to the one that has cared for them thus far. These intrepid travelers are not rare. This chapter does not address the issues of the medical traveler coming to the United States seeking health care. That broad topic is related but is not the subject of this section. The medical evacuation and medical assistance programs available for repatriation will be given only short coverage. The focus of this chapter is the emerging resources of electronic information and telecommunications to support the traveler with regard to health needs. Electronic information and telecommunications applied to health care define telemedicine. No matter where you are, you should be in an electronic continuum with familiar, competent, and interactive health care.

Health needs abroad are usually thought of as traveler's diarrhea, other infectious diseases, and injuries. However, our infirmities travel with us, and we travel with increasing frequency. Unexpected health challenges may arise in travel. However, many people are also engaged in vigorous programs of disease management, and they bring along not only the imponderable risk of accident but also the daily need to manage a chronic condition. What risks do those with health issues really take in international travel? What are the resources that might help them? What preparations before travel are prudent and practical? In this brief chapter, the scope of medical issues in travel will be considered along with the comparative anatomy of health services in the United States and abroad. Most important, the excellent resources in telecommunications and electronic information will be reviewed along with those services that the public demands and the steadily improving technology may bring to bear in the near future. Ideally, our medical care should be as portable as our medical conditions.

The Problem

There is much commentary about the graying of America. The average age in the United States is 35.3 years, having increased 17.7% in the last 20 years.[2] Life expectancy has risen from 73.7 to 76.9 years in the last 20 years. Compare that with the average life expectancy of 47.3 years in 1900.[3,4] This has significant implications for travel. There are many older Americans in retirement, with the time and resources to travel. However, of the 61 million Americans who went abroad last year, 15 million were on business trips, with the average age of the traveler being 47 years.[5,6] That traveling work force is aging and, like the general population, will not be replaced by a surge of 20-somethings anxious to take on the exciting work opportunities abroad. Approximately 4 million Americans live and work abroad at least 3 months per year, and they now increasingly include employees over 50 who are involved in construction, finance, and education.[7]

The overall increase in age means that the worker or traveler carries along the expected degenerative diseases and risks for health crisis. The hotel doctor well known in travel books may not be enough. The traveler/patient may need clarification about a medication, a medication reaction, or a symptom best addressed by the personal physician back home. More serious health crises entail a call to 911 rather than a friendly visit by the hotel physician. There is an incorrect assumption that questions about health problems are handled about the same way in all countries. Even in the many parts of the world where health care is excellent, the logistics of health care may be almost as exotic as the local language or cuisine. The ways a society molds medicine to its needs is a complicated process of sociology, economics, and prevailing resources. It is fair to say that there is no country in the world that approaches healthcare delivery in the same way as the United States. Frankly, no other country really wants to use our approach even if money was not the issue! We are marvelously eccentric in addition to having very advanced services available with relative ease. Relative ease of access does not imply that we are the paragon of health care. However, when abroad we cannot expect familiar approaches to medical care.

In the United States, we generally utilize a primary care physician who keeps rather good paper or electronic records of our care. The physician's office is available most of the time; after hours, an answering service will find someone capable of responding to our questions and problems. Most physicians participate in contracting arrangements with our insurance coverage, and we see our primary care physicians and specialists in a system that requires us to keep the insurance coverage current, pay part of the medical bill as a co-pay, and, if we need urgent hospitalization or are away from home and need urgent care, our insurance carriers have a way to cover our services. Our insurance coverage does not necessarily travel abroad, where access to hospitals is usually quite separate from access to physicians' offices.

Prescriptions are often covered with a small payment in the United States. The records are kept in such a way as to make refills fairly easy, and communication with physicians is fairly generous. The distribution of drugs is carefully regulated, and the cost is rather high. But prescription refills abroad can be a nightmare. Our personal physicians are not readily available, and even if they were, they are not licensed to practice in another country. The names of the drugs may be very different, and doses are not uniform throughout the world. English is not always spoken and medical practice including details of treatment may be at sharp variance with what we know from home. This does not mean that the diagnostic procedures or treatments are wrong; they are just different, and medical encounters may rapidly deteriorate into distrust and confusion.

When a crisis arises during travel, your hotel or your country's consulate can help you find a physician who speaks English. If you need hospitalization, you may be a candidate for air evacuation to a country with definitive care or for repatriation back to the United States. These emergencies are handled rather well, but the care is very expensive.[8,9]

E-Health Solutions

What are the e-health resources available to aid the traveler as a potential or actual patient? In fact, the resources are numerous but underutilized. Let us start with the individual traveler. Patients, traveling or stationary, need not be passive with regard to their health or illness. A little self-knowledge and personal responsibility can greatly influence health and determine the outcome of disease management. The notion of the patient in charge, informed, and in partnership with health care has grown from tentative aspiration to reality in recent years. Therefore, you should be able to explain your medical situation to a new doctor even in a very different healthcare environment.

For example, you should know your blood type, past medical history, past surgical history, and any history of drug allergies. This knowledge allows you to concisely interact with a health facility should the need arise. If you are on a medication, you should know the name of the medicine, the dose, and the purpose. Memory need not be trusted. You can request from your primary care physician a medical summary and drug list. Medications are marketed by different names in other countries so generic names can be useful in communication with health personnel abroad because those names are applied universally. If you are managing hypertension, diabetes, or a heart rhythm abnormality, you should know and have with you the blood pressure pattern, lab values, and EKG tracings, which are being monitored should a problem arise while traveling. In fact, a visit to your primary care physician for advice and review prior to travel could have real merit.

Travel clinics in most U.S. cities can advise you about the specific area of travel in your plan and the pitfalls or possibilities of that particular area. These clinics can advise about immunizations, infection risks, food problems, water issues, etc. They may also prescribe certain medications to have on hand should problems arise, such as traveler's diarrhea. Travel medicine even has a name as a medical specialty: emporiatrics. Dr. Mary Nettlemen's book, by the same title, has a wonderful reference list of print resources about traveler's health. Portable medical records, informed travelers, emporiatrics, and emergency resource information sum up what could be done in even the recent past with regard to travel. With these four tools, a journey could begin with all the preparation that was possible before the advent of cyberspace.

A search of the Web by almost any engine can overwhelm even the most determinedly curious. There are millions of pages of medical information, which resist reduction by even the best key word user. However, some sites are easily recommended. The U.S. State Department (http://www.state.gov/travel) gives the medical traveler excellent health information by country. The State Department site also lists the phone numbers of the U.S. embassy in your destination country and the nearest consulate should your itinerary take you outside the national capital. Write that down or put it in your personal digital assistant (PDA) for quick reference. The local consulate or consular section of the embassy is a great resource for directions to competent health care. Remember, the diplomats and their dependents are experts because they may have needed these services themselves. They know which doctors speak English, have U.S. credentials, and have been helpful to travelers before. The World Health Organization describes health statistics and health resources in various countries (http://www.who.int/ith/). Travelers can also check the latest health information with the U.S. Centers for Disease Control and Prevention (http://www.cdc.gov/travel/index.htm) for additional traveler's health information. The Web sites for individual nations usually describe health resources, clinics, and issues for travelers. For example, Madagascar's Web site (http://www.embassy.org/madagascar/) lists specific vaccination recommendations and health risks such as malaria or crocodile bite! The International Association for Medical Assistance to Travelers (http://www.iamat.org/) has a list of recommended hospitals or clinics for travelers abroad.

Use the Yellow Pages to find a travel clinic before you leave, or check the Web site for the International Society of Travel Medicine (http://www.istm.org/), which identifies travel medicine practitioners and clinics operated by its members by location. If you know in advance that you must see a physician for laboratory monitoring or other reasons while you're away, work with your physician and employer and perhaps the hotel at your destination to make the contact ahead of time. The International Association for Medical Advice to Travelers (http://www.iamat.org/) provides a list of English-speaking physicians meeting minimum requirements. The American Board of Medical Specialties (ABMS) Web site (http://www.abms.org/) can tell you which physicians in a variety of countries have U.S. credentials, and the ABMS publication "The Official ABMS Directory of Board Certified Specialists" lists specialists who practice in the place you are visiting. These physicians have trained in the United States in the same programs as U.S. health providers and should be comfortable interacting with U.S. patients.

If you have a PDA, you should record your medical history and medical issues or notes. The PDA can store information about international clinics, embassies, etc. It has ample memory to keep all the data you might need. If your medical history is lengthy, perhaps storage on a disk would be better. You can even have critical x-ray studies put on a CD that you can take with you, which could save repetition of studies or provide a basis for precise comparison should something in your condition change.

Once you assemble your medical history, record it electronically, and make it portable, you now own an electronic medical record. The Kennedy-Kassebaum act of 1996 called for a national medical record in the United States. Concerns about privacy led to cancellation of the plan in 1997. But the idea continues to have such merit that the U.S. military uses an electronic record that can be carried around like a credit card. It is ironic that we have magnetic strips that make us known at ATMs around the world and can get money in Marrakech, baubles in Bali, and rugs in Rangoon, but you cannot get your prescription refilled until you return home.

Travel for work or pleasure traditionally allows little more than a postcard to report home, and the card frequently takes longer to get home than the traveler. With some effort a long-distance phone call can be made. However, current technology makes that sort of incognito voyage only pertinent to those who really need to be incognito! Be sure you have the phone number of your personal physician and take along a phone card with the access number for the country you are visiting. Be sure you have the fax number of your doctor. You should also have emergency notification information readily available. Phone service around the world is usually better than travelers expect, and pleasant surprises may be in store. Travel may be more exotic in the many parts of the planet with poor phone service or no Internet access. Should you need contact with your physician for monitoring, an iridium satellite phone is not hard to carry. At a cost of $1,000 the phone can connect you to home. Monitoring devices can be connected to your laptop computer and data sent by iridium phone as well.[10-13] Soon these data, voice, and video connections will be readily handled by cellular phone or interactive PDA.[14-16]

There is no reason to cease being a prudent medical consumer of e-health while away. Internet access from your hotel, workplace, Internet café, or by modem with your own computer are all realistic. If you have a health question, go to the same source you would use at home, such as WebMD (http://webmd.com/). The site is available wherever there is an Internet connection. If you are used to seeking medical information from the National Library of Medicine (http://www.nlm.nih.gov/) or National Institutes of Health (http://www.nih.gov/) or the Web sites of major medical centers like the Mayo Clinic (http://www.mayo.edu/) or Johns Hopkins (http://www.hopkinsmedicine.org/), their Web sites are just a click away. Should you have trouble with a disease management issue, log on to the Web site of the disease in question, such as the American Diabetes Association (http://www.diabetes.org/), American Heart Association (http://www.americanheart.org/), Crohn's disease (http://www.crohnsresource.com/), or the International Ostomy Society (http://www.ostomyinternational.org/), and continue the habit of participating in your own health care no matter where you are. Perhaps your personal physician's staff will want you to use their e-mail address to report your blood pressure, glucose, or weight. You may even have an arrangement to check your pacemaker or heart rhythm by phone while you are away. The objective is to weave an electronic connection among you, your physician, your family, and the resources at hand wherever you travel. That connection permits travel with confidence and much greater safety.

As an informed medical consumer, further resources to care for you as a tourist or worker abroad will depend in many ways on what you demand. Let us consider a few emerging services. Most aircraft and cruise ships now have some arrangement for telemedicine consultation. What is telemedicine? Broadly, it is the use of telecommunications to support health care over distances.[17] In the instance of air or sea travelers, it is the ability to seek expert medical advice to assess emergencies. International telemedicine services may also be available in your destination country. Approximately 400,000 Americans require emergency medical assistance while traveling abroad each year.[9] With aging or ailing travelers, these services become all the more necessary.

MEDJET Assistance (http://www.medjetassistance.com/) is one of a number of companies that provide worldwide air medical evacuation and emergency consultation services that are available 24 hours a day, 7 days a week.

Your company may have arrangements for telemedicine services with videoconference, consultation, arrangements for air evacuation, or local treatment. One such service, MedAire, Inc. (http://www.medaire.com/), logged 8526 calls in 2000. Aviation telemedicine is provided on a global basis to commercial airlines, business jets, maritime operators, and government agencies alike. Similar to the airline industry, the cruise ship industry has healthcare guidelines for cruise ship medical facilities as well. These guidelines were created by the American College of Emergency Physicians and have been incorporated by the International Council of Cruise Lines (http://www.acep.org/1,593,0.html).

The equipment to monitor medical conditions gets more portable all the time, and digital measurements can be easily transmitted to your managing physician no matter where you are. Siemens Medical Solutions, Inc. (http://www.siemensmedical.com/) is making great strides in disease management and screening services for chronic diseases. Their DIADEM (Diabetes Disease Management) project, which studies type 2 diabetes, hopes to have Europe-wide services within the next few years with eventual international availability. The Information Society Technologies TOSCA project (http://tosca.gsf.de/) is working to establish a telescreening system with the goal of reducing blindness caused by diabetic retinopathy and glaucoma. Wireless EKG monitoring by telephone has proven successful in several research studies and the hope is for EKG screening to be made widely acceptable and simplified for home use. Therefore, it is possible for your personal physician to participate in your care no matter where you are through proper telecommunications.

With the use of a "smart card" like the ones manufactured by Gemplus (http://www.gemplus.com/) and the Universal-ID card (http://www.universal-id.com/), you can have your entire medical history available at any time to support your care. Smart cards are credit-card sized plastic cards with an embedded computer chip. An entire medical history can fit neatly into a wallet.

In a time of unprecedented mobility, there is no justification for distance to compromise health or disease management. A well-informed medical consumer using the best resources today and demanding the best resources for tomorrow will steadily raise the standards of e-health.

References

1. Center on an Aging Society. Institute for Health Care Research and Policy, Georgetown University, Data Profile Number 5, September 2002. http://ihcrp.georgetown.edu/agingsociety/rxdrugs/rxdrugs.html.
2. U.S. Census Bureau. Census 2000 profile of general demographic characteristics for the United States: 2000 and 1980 census of population, vol 1, characteristics of the population (PC80-1). Washington, DC: U.S. Census Bureau, 1980, 2000.
3. National Center for Health Statistics. National Vital Statistic Rep 2001;49(12); 2002;50(6).
4. Centers for Disease Control. Ten great public health achievements: about a century of success. October 2002. http://www.phppo.cdc.gov/PHTN/tenachievements/about/about1.asp

5. U.S. Department of Commerce, International Trade Administration. http://www.tinet.ita.doc.gov/research/reports.
6. HTH Worldwide, Inc. http://www.hthbusiness.com/faq.cfm.
7. American Citizens Abroad. http://www.aca.ch/
8. MedAire, Inc. http://www.medaire.com/
9. MEDJET Assistance. http://www.medjetassistance.com/longway.asp?partner=ild
10. Doarn CR, Fitzgerald S, Rodas E, Harnett B, Merrell RC. Telemedicine to integrate intermittent surgical services into primary care. Telemed J and e-Health 2002;8(1):131–137.
11. Broderick TJ, Harnett BM, Merriam NR, Kapoor V, Doarn CR, Merrell RC. Impact of varying transmission bandwidth on image quality in laparoscopic telemedicine. Telemed J and e-Health 2001;7(1):47–53.
12. Angood P, Harnett B, Merriam N, Satava R, Doarn CR, Merrell RC. The benefits of integrating Internet technology with standard communications for telemedicine in extreme environments. Aviat Space Environ Med 2001;72(12):1132–1137.
13. Satava RM, Angood PB, Harnett BM, Merrell RC. The physiologic cipher at altitude: telemedicine and real-time monitoring of climbers on Mount Everest. Telemed J 2000;6(3):303–313.
14. Orlov OI, Drozdov DV, Doarn CR, Merrell RC. Wireless ECG monitoring by telephone leads. Telemed J E Health 2000;7(1):33–38.
15. Harnett BM, Doarn CR, Russell KM, Kapoor V, Merriam NR, Merrell RC. Wireless telemetry and Internet technologies for medical management: a Martian analogy. Aviat Space Environ Med 2001;72(12):1125–1131.
16. Rosser JC, Bell RL, Harnett BM, Rodas E, Murayama M, Merrell RC. Use of mobile low-bandwidth telemedical techniques for extreme telemedicine application. Am Coll Surg J 1999;189(4):397–404.
17. The Institute of Medicine, Field M, ed. Telemedicine: a guide to assessing telecommunications in health care. Washington, DC: National Academy Press, 1996.

Epilogue: Power to the Patient

DAVID ELLIS

Consumer informatics in health care is a blend of health-, clinical-, and bio-informatics. As the lines between them grow blurred, the combination is destined to grow into the central edifice of all health care. Whether at the public health level or an individual's proteome level, biology and medicine have become a numbers game, with numbers to describe our genome and numbers to guide diagnostic, therapeutic, and augmentative technologies.

Numbers are computable, and increasingly powerful computers crunch an exponentially growing number of numbers as we explore and create ever more complex systems. At the same time, the falling costs, smaller size, and growing ease of use of computer devices put more number-crunching diagnostic and therapeutic capacity into the hands of ordinary healthcare consumers. I have presented forecasts of the trends in computing capacity elsewhere.[1] In this epilogue, on the basis that the future of consumer health informatics is, in a growing real sense, the future of health care, I seek to extend the discussion to forecasting the consequences of the numbers-based and informatics-based innovations in healthcare technologies. First, a word about long-term forecasting; then, a forecast.

Long-Term Forecasting

I'm not sure whether to be alarmed or encouraged that more and more quite respectable people are starting to venture out with me onto the thin ice of trend forecasting, making projections based on historical trend data about the power and capabilities of technologies, and pointing to potential consequences. UCLA professor Gregory Stock,[2] for example, is out there, too, forecasting that genetic engineering could eliminate disease, confer near-immortality, and redesign the human being. These would be stunning leaps, indeed. But in general, as reviewer Tom Abate notes, "Advances only appear to be stunning leaps to those who haven't paid attention," and he encourages us to pay more attention to incremental advances.[3] He shudders (as I do, though perhaps for different reasons) at Stock's belief in the ultimate goodness of free markets and his forecast that wealthy parents will pay for better babies. Abate is rightly concerned that futurists (possibly including myself) are too quick to classify a small step as a huge leap. He points out, as have others, that although the mapping of the human genome has increased our knowledge of the causes of health and disease, it has nevertheless posed more questions than it has produced answers. The trick of long-term forecasting, it seems to me, is to identify the particular small steps that harbinger the stunning leap.

In vitro fertilization and embryo screening technologies, for example, which already enable parents to choose the sex of their child, or screen out a diseased one, seemed a stunning leap at the time, but in retrospect were just a harbinger of in vitro and in utero genetic engineering of "designer babies." Scientists have already engineered mice embryos to produce translucent green mice with better memories.[4] Evolution is "satisfied"[a] with whatever is "good enough" for survival of the species, but we demand survival of the individual. The phenotype has begun to dominate the genotype, and is teaching the selfish gene a lesson.

The passivity of the current processes of fertilization and screening enervates their ethics, but they are on their way to becoming active processes where the ethics scream loud if not always clear. Ethics would seem to be one good reason for making forecasts about the longer-term technologies and their consequences, but in the end, are they not a future generation's problem? Well, yes and no. Yes, because (if Stock and I and other futurists don't fall through the ice with our predictions of longevity) we *are* that future generation. No, because according to my special theory of relativity for innovations, as innovation accelerates, it expands the space we experience at any given moment, by revealing or creating areas of the cosmos and of the microcosm previously inaccessible, unknown, or nonexistent. Correspondingly, time contracts in inverse proportion to the expansion of our speed through the new space. Acceleration in healthcare innovation is such that the longer term has contracted from a hundred years as perceived by early 20th century observers, to 10 years as perceived by early 21st century observers, and it is shrinking. Ten years is time enough to make a difference to almost every current generation, including the aging Baby Boomers.

The TV science fiction series "Star Trek" explores and sometimes offers interesting insights into the long-term future. Yet its scriptwriters seem to have their heads in the Magellanic clouds and are missing what is happening on

---

[a]Satisfice: "To obtain an outcome that is good enough. Satisficing action can be contrasted with maximising action, which seeks the biggest, or with optimising action, which seeks the best. In recent decades doubts have arisen about the view that in all rational decision-making the agent seeks the best result. Instead, it is argued, it is often rational to seek to satisfice i.e. to get a good result that is good enough although not necessarily the best. The term was introduced by Herbert A. Simon in his Models of Man 1957." Source: Mautner T, ed. *The Penguin Dictionary of Philosophy.*

planet Earth. Take their idea of cyborgism, as represented by the amoral, soulless "Borg," for example. The Borg is a hive-like society of interconnected cyborgs¾part-biological, part-machine beings whose main aim in life is to assimilate other species. Technologically, the notion is sound. Cyborgs already exist: check out David Beresford's report on his life as a cyborg after having an electronic device implanted into his brain to control the symptoms of Parkinson's disease.[5] But except for a blind character fitted with a sight-giving eyeglasses-like device, "Star Trek" appears to miss the beneficial side and the fact of human progress toward cyborgism.[b]

Perhaps this is because the scriptwriter cannot know what the possibilities are without experiencing cyborgism at first hand—the philosopher's "What is it like to be a bat?" problem.[6] It is easier to write stories about our own species, or those around us, than about aliens; about the familiar and known, than about the unfamiliar or unknown. Even the Borg are presented in a form familiar to us—just your everyday amoral, uncaring, seekers of power who just happen, in this case, to be part-machine. But technological innovations are helping answer the philosopher's question, and have shown us, for example, what it is like to be able to communicate instantly with almost anyone, almost anytime, almost anywhere via cell phones and the Internet. This was hard (though not impossible) to imagine before cell phones and the Internet. Such innovations force scriptwriters, without their knowing it, to write different scripts. The hit 1967 movie *The Graduate*, for example, would need to be radically rewritten as a contemporary movie, because its upper-middle-class characters would all have cell phones, rendering unnecessary the long, suspenseful scenes where the hero drives around town in frantic search of a phone booth, begs for coins to make a call, and prays that his heroine will be home when her phone rings.[7] Today's scripts, which routinely include cell phones if calls are to be made, will not work for future movies where characters will routinely possess brain implants for telepathic communication via the wireless Internet. My point is that scriptwriters of the reality movie *Health Care 2020* ought not to be basing their policy and strategy scripts on 2002 technologies; they need to use their imaginations rather more than they have been accustomed to so far.

For instance, what will healthcare strategists and policymakers of today do to prepare for the projected 157 million chronically ill patients by 2020?[8] With just six chronic conditions (asthma, heart disease, diabetes, back conditions, depression, and kidney failure) already accounting for 30% of employers' health care dollars[8] (not to mention for an awful lot of human pain and suffering), it is natural and right to worry and to take preventive or palliative action. But it would be wrong to despair about the long term and make desperate decisions affecting it, when the trends forecast cures for most if not all chronic conditions by then. We have already found a cure for osteoporosis in postmeno-

---

[b] Not being a fanatical "Trekkie," I have not seen every episode and may have missed some discussion of the issue, but my point is that the writers ignored cyborgism as a fundamental component of the future and of every human crew member.

pausal women, and for men with primary or hypogonadal osteoporosis,[c] as well as a vaccine for cervical cancer,[9] and we are on the verge of cures for other forms of cancer, diabetes, malaria (not an American disease, but huge world-wide), Alzheimer's, cardiovascular disease, and others. Disease prevalence projections need to be accompanied by the economist's caveat: *ceteris paribus*—"other things being equal." The acceleration of innovations guaran-tees that *ceteris* will not be *paribus*; and it will be dangerous to base healthcare strategies and policy on long-term projections that do not take accelerating technology trends into account.

Of all technological trends, none will have as great a consequence as that toward increasing autonomy in machines.

Decision Support, Machine Autonomy

The Mars polar lander crashed in 1999, because its computers could not handle false sensor readings. That same year, Deep Space One also suffered an unex-pected misfortune yet survived to tell the tale of the asteroid it was sent to meet. The difference was that the surviving craft had "model-based reason-ing" capability, allowing it to know when something was wrong and to figure out a fix.[10] This is not "Star Trek"; this is real.

Autonomy is needed where human control is impossible or undesirable, and that does not just mean in outer space. It means wherever complexity is so great as to overwhelm the human brain's capacity. Such complexity exists in the computerized systems that run our automobiles, office equipment, and databases, not to mention heating, ventilation, and air-conditioning systems, telephone and computer networks, air traffic control systems, and power sta-tions and grids. It also exists, we are now discovering, in the human genome and, orders of magnitude below that, in the proteome.

Model-based reasoning is a deceptively simple approach to writing reliable decision-making programs for systems growing too complex for the human mind to grasp in their entirety. The only thing the system architect needs to anticipate is the desired end result—a soft landing on Mars, say; while the model-based reasoning system works out the actual details of what to do to achieve that human-set goal.

Robert Morris, director of IBM's Almaden Research Center in San Jose, CA, said, "We spend so much of our time managing ... systems and so much of our money paying people to run them. We'd better stop spending so much on the tedium and more on the new technologies."[10] The main tedium to be overcome is the skepticism of unimaginative humans, who would be wise either to get out of the way of the technological tsunami of innovation or, like the under-

---

[c] The drug is Forteo; see its maker Eli Lilly's press release at http://newsroom.lilly.com/news/story.cfm?ID=1143.

standably risk-averse NASA mission managers who did not at first want to trust the fate of Deep Space One to a model-based reasoning system, to climb onto their surfboards and ride the wave. Success breeds confidence (and failures such as the Mars polar lander breed the opposite), and autonomous, model-based reasoning systems will be widely adopted in health care as elsewhere, when we have eliminated the tedium. To those with the will and the means to surf the tsunami of machine autonomy, the result will be a new and exhilarating level of empowerment.

Patient Empowerment

The Patient Centered Access to Secure Systems Online (PCASSO) electronic medical record project was "a true vanguard in patient empowerment" (see Chapter 5). Patient empowerment is a key element of the trend to patient self-care. Cynics are right to warn of a hidden message: "You're on your own, pal,"[11] but the day is coming when being on one's own in health care will be perfectly OK; when one is fully empowered not just to manage one's own care, but to provide it also—to be physician and surgeon. Through small, harbinger steps like PCASSO, patient empowerment technology will reach the level of the "Star Trek" "tricorder," which, with a noninvasive wave over the patient, diagnoses and fixes everything. We are well on our way to such a device, with existing tools of empowerment including the following:

1. Information technologies, including Web sites, Internet communications (e-mail, instant messaging, Web conferencing), portals, telehealth (videoconferencing)
2. Disease management technologies, including a longitudinal PCASSO-like EMR and online access to management assistance offered by care providers and health plans
3. Assistive technologies, including robotic aides and prostheses
4. Monitoring and diagnostic technologies, including handheld, wearable, or implanted devices for telehealth telemetry
5. Therapeutic technologies, including inhalers, nanomedical "Qdot" or dendrimer injections or smart pills, stem cell transplants, and genetic/proteomic engineering

These are not "Star Trek," either; they are real.

The better technology becomes at contributing to patient care, the less the patient or physician needs to be an active, conscious, directing participant spending time making decisions about what to do. Taking the doctor and the patient out of the loop assumes autonomous, sensitive, intelligent machines able to assess our state of health and make decisions accordingly. We see the development of just such capabilities in the extraordinary artificial intelligence (AI) entities that populate computer games such as "Black and White."[d] But it may not be necessary to have a superintelligent AI entity to maintain health.

Injectable "Qdots" (nanoscale "quantum dots" wrapped in protein peptides that home to specific addresses inside living tissue—a breast cancer, for example—without causing blood clotting to choke off the blood supply and thereby kill the tumor)[12] are not intelligent, but they know where to go and what do in a given circumstance, and that may be enough.

Consequences of Innovations

A consequence of increasing technology autonomy is that physicians will have less and less impact on consumer's choice of drugs as drug companies more and more market directly to the consumer on an individualized, and eventually genome-customized, basis. It is a good bet (projecting the trend line) that by 2008, people will be able to have their own genomes inexpensively and quickly sequenced through a new generation of automated gene sequencers now in development. The first-generation automated sequencers read about 5000 base pairs per day. Today's machines sequence about a million bases a day. DNA microarrays can now detect millions of sequences at a time. US Genomics has developed a machine that scans a single DNA molecule 200,000 bases long in milliseconds and aims to sequence the genome no slower than "instantaneously."[13]

What will we do with our personal genome maps? In the short term, we may simply shop them around and invite physicians to fix a genetic anomaly. In the long term, our personal digital physician may reengineer our genome on the fly to suit a given purpose or environment.

The current generation of medical devices includes cardiac pacemakers, implantable drug-infusion pumps, blood sugar monitors worn like a wrist watch, brain pacemakers for Parkinson's sufferers,[5] wound dressings made of manufactured skin, a bionic retina, semiautonomous robotic prosthetic limbs, an artificial pancreas, drug-coated stents, videocam capsules that take pictures as they pass through the digestive tract, and an implanted ID/medical record chip. Who checks these things out before they are unleashed on patients? In the United States, it is the Food and Drug Administration (FDA). And therein lies a problem—the problem of the acceleration of innovations. The U.S. House of Representatives passed a bill in October 2002 to help the FDA speed its approval of such devices.[14] Evidently the government is being forced by the acceleration of innovations to accelerate its own processes. Whether it will be able to keep pace is another matter. Going from the current 400 days to the proposed 300 days may be a large percentage drop, but 300 days is still almost a year, and the special theory of relativity in innovation is likely to render the bill moot. A year is a decade in "Internet time," and envelope-pushing compa-

---

[d] For a good review of the state of the art in games, see Steven Johnson, "Wild Things." *Wired*, October 10, 2002. http://www.wired.com/wired/archive/10.03/aigames.html.

nies like Verichip will probably not sit idly by while the fruit of their investment withers on the vine and foreign competitors steal their markets.

The message of the medium of individually empowering, and therefore liberating, technologies is individual empowerment and individual independence. Through the 19th and 20th centuries we handed over much of our independence to people who knew how to control technologies. The farmer with his tractor dictated what we would eat; the locomotive engineer and airplane pilot and their schedulers, how we would get from A to B, and when; the broadcast TV moguls, what we would see on TV; and the doctor, how we would regain or retain good health.

Technology gave these experts the edge, because technology was then complex to use. I first learned to drive in a car with a nonsynchronous gearbox, which meant I had to "double de-clutch" whenever changing gears, and on a downshift I had to rev the engine between the de-clutches. In general, the simpler the technology, the more difficult it is to use. My car today has a much more complex automatic gearbox, but I am almost oblivious of it. It takes care of the gearing and clutching for me.

Even as we benefit from it so obviously, and even as our initial distrust dissolves the instant we experience the benefits (as we have in automatic gearboxes and model-based reasoning systems in spacecraft, printers, and automobiles), we intuitively fight, or conspicuously ignore, the trend to machine control. Leading nanomedicine theorist Robert Freitas "argues for diagnostic and therapeutic 'gatekeeping' by a single *trusted* [my emphasis] practitioner in whom strategic treatment responsibility is vested—in partnership, of course, with the patient."[15] We leap upon a single failure, such as the death of Barney Clark or the crash of an early-model Airbus when its automated "fly-by-wire" controls overrode the pilot's efforts to avert disaster, as we tend to leap upon the lone swallow and declare it is summer. But that distrust does not stop us from putting our car into automatic gear and leaving the house with the gas oven timed to cook dinner at 450 degrees unattended for our return, or drooling over the automated, drive-by-wire autos Detroit is about to roll out, or hoping that Abiocor will have perfected its artificial heart by the time we need one ourselves.

The risk inherent in trusting our oven timer is orders of magnitude smaller than the risk inherent to trusting the automated, autonomous nuclear power plant next door, or the visiting robo-surgeon, or an artificial heart, and it is right that we insist these autonomous devices be rigorously tested before being unleashed on humanity. But it is wrong to ignore them, because they are inevitable and they will make a great difference in our lives, for the better. All modern jetliners are now automated, fly-by-wire aircraft, à l'Airbus.

Nevertheless, optimism about the wonderful consequences of the technologies of the future must be tempered by the fact that the healthcare system today is an acknowledged mess. The anticipation of cures for chronic diseases is no excuse for not *immediately* raising the quality of care, reducing its costs, and extending its benefits to all people. We must begin to pay more than lip service to evidence-based medicine and use the tools innovation has already delivered (the Internet for sharing evidence, databases for storing it, and decision-support systems for acting on it). I doubt that intelligent, autonomous, personal digital physicians will be as reticent as physicians appear to have been to embrace evidence-based medicine. I hope my PDP will not hesitate to contact its colleagues worldwide to gather and assess all available relevant information about a cure or enhancement for its patient.

In 1947 IBM chairman Tom Watson estimated a world market for "maybe five" computers. Apparently, his power of prediction was no better nearly two decades later: In 1965, he said that electronic medical records would be widespread in "just a few years."[16] In the first case, he failed to see that there *was* a need; in the second case, he failed to see that there was *not* a need, as far as the provider market was concerned. His first forecast was a failure of vision, but not his second. The second was a failure of implementation, because the real market—the patient—was not consulted.[e]

No matter whether the "Star Trek" doctor was human, alien, or hologram, he betrayed his scriptwriter's failure of vision. A holographic doctor is unrealistic, not because of the concept that an artificially intelligent computer with a projected hologram interface can represent a person (a reasonable proposition), but because of the concept that tricorder-equipped people will continue to be passive, unempowered patients for centuries to come, which is patently preposterous.

Let's hope our health care scriptwriters get the message.

References

1. Ellis D. Technology and the future of health care: preparing for the next 30 years. San Francisco: Jossey-Bass, 2000.
2. Stock G. Redesigning humans: our inevitable genetic future. 2002.
3. Abate T. "Designer baby" proponent to address biotech investors. San Francisco Chronicle, October 21, 2002, p. E-1.
4. Coghlan A. Genetic modification alters hair colour. New Scientist, September 9, 2002. http://www.newscientist.com/news/news.jsp?id=ns99992774, citing Proceedings of the National Academy of Sciences (DOI: /10.1073/pnas.192453799).
5. Beresford D. My life as a cyborg. The Guardian, December 3, 2002. http://www.guardian.co.uk/medicine/story/0,11381,852542,00.html.
6. Nagel T. "What is it like to be a bat?" Philosophical Review 1974;83(4):435–450.
7. National Public Radio. NPR: cell phones and movies. 2002. Sound file available at http://discover.npr.org/rundowns/segment.jhtml?wfId=863809.
8. Walker M. Kaiser challenge: how to manage chronic disease. San Francisco Business Times, October 18, 2002.

[e]But it is beginning to be consulted. I am involved in an EMR initiative in Michigan that puts patients at the center and that actively seeks patient support, not just provider support.

9. Koutsky LA, et al. A controlled trial of a human papillomavirus type 16 vaccine. N Engl J Med 2002;347:1645–1651.

10. Roush W. Immobots take control. Technol Rev December 2002/January 2003. http://www.technologyreview.com/articles/roush1202.asp

11. Morrison I. Wary of choices. Health Forum J 2002;45(5):48.

12. BBC. High tech tattoos. 2002. http://news.bbc.co.uk/2/hi/health/2225404.stm.

13. Westphal SP. Race for the $1000 genome is on. New Scientist 2002. http://www.newscientist.com/news/news.jsp?id=ns99992900

14. H.R.5651. http://thomas.loc.gov.

15. Weber DO. The next little thing. Health Forum J 2002;45(5):12.

16. Willenson M. Demanding medical excellence: doctors and accountability in the Information Age. Chicago: University of Chicago Press, 1999:359.

Index

Health Informatics Series
(formerly Computers in Health Care)

(continued from page ii)

Medical Informatics
Computer Applications in Health Care and Biomedicine, Second Edition
E.H. Shortliffe and L.E. Perreault

Filmless Radiology
E.L. Siegel and R.M. Kolodner

Cancer Informatics
Essential Technologies for Clinical Trials
J.S. Silva, M.J. Ball, C.G. Chute, J.V. Douglas, C.P. Langlotz, J.C. Niland, and W.L. Scherlis

Clinical Information Systems
A Component-Based Approach
R. Van de Velde and P. Degoulet

Knowledge Coupling
New Premises and New Tools for Medical Care and Education
L.L. Weed